WHY HENRY VIII GOT FAT

Why Henry VIII *got* FAT

SECRETS WE CAN DISCOVER ABOUT WEIGHT-LOSS FROM FAMOUS 'BIG' PEOPLE

MIA CAMPBELL

FREE GIFT

To thank you for your purchase and time, I'm offering a free quiz & guide to help you discover your unique health personality.

In *Your Health Personality*, you'll learn about 4 health personalities and find out which one is most like you. Then you'll see which eating habits and exercises could work best for you.

Discovering your health personality could help you make better, more lasting choices that will help your life and health in many ways. You could also find out why other lifestyle changes haven't worked for you in the past.

Go to the link below to download it free:

http://yourhealthpersonality. subscribemenow.com

I hope you enjoy it.

Mia

ALSO BY MIA CAMPBELL

The 10-Day Skin Brushing Detox

Inversion Therapy

For Deborah Howard,
in memory of your lovely Mum

Contents

Introduction

Why My Quest Started With Henry

I've been fascinated with the glamorous Tudor period since my schooldays. I wrote a little play set in the era, that my class put on. We all dressed up in colorful curtains instead of Tudor gowns but we felt fabulous!

I'm not alone. There are thousands of people, all over the world, who are as obsessed with the Tudors as I am. Countless websites, clubs, societies, and reenactment groups abound. What is it with that era?

Their lives were full of mystery, intrigue, danger, and daring ... and they wore fabulous clothes! They were the 16th century equivalent of today's celebrities. Tabloid fodder, avidly snapped up by a waiting populace. But these were real A-list celebs, not reality TV ones, and Henry had massive power – deadly power.

We are fascinated by stories of Henry's excesses – his daring (for a prince) hobbies and athleticism, his eating habits, the number of his wives, the number of people he had killed, the terrifying decisions he made that still have an impact on his country today.

The Tudor period was one of wild scandal and startling excess. It fascinated and horrified the world then and it still does, 400 years later. Just as the tabloids are mesmerized by Kim Kardashian's rear end, we are spellbound by Henry's massive girth. The press takes great interest in celebrity fashions – they always have. The press of Henry's day were interested in his clothing and historians are glad they were, as we have been left with accurate records of Henry's measurements and how they increased over time.

It's because I'm such a Tudor freak that I will read or watch anything and everything that is about them and that period. One of the things that really fascinated me was a National Geographic documentary on TV a while back called *Inside the body of Henry VIII*[1].

It was described as a 'virtual autopsy'. A team of experts looked at Henry's history – medical, physical, emotional, and everything else. It was fascinating, as it showed the effects Henry's accidents and eating habits had on his body.

I also found it a little worrying. Like Henry, I had an accident that stopped my sporting and active hobbies; it also gave me a similar concussion. Also like him, I started putting weight on after my accident.

---

[1]   http://channel.nationalgeographic.com/channel/episodes/inside-the-body-of-henry-viii/

I wanted to learn more about Henry's massive weight gain and that led me to research other obese people from history to see if there was a common thread. There are several threads. There are things that are common to people with weight issues.

My research and writing of this book has turned my feelings about dieting on their head. I'm a qualified aromatherapist and my training and additional post-qualification studies included nutrition and anatomy & physiology. I thought I was clued up about stuff like this. But I have still fallen, over the years, for dieting and health fads.

I did a one week juice fast that was very successful. I lost 11lbs in that week and I felt great. Until I started eating again. I ended up in hospital with gallbladder problems.

It made me reconsider the wisdom of fasting and that was confirmed when I started looking at the life stories of the people who feature in this book. Most of them tried fasting and crash diets and most of them ruined their health through them.

My late mother-in-law, Elsie, was once very large. She lost all her excess weight and never regained it. She managed it because an ex-ballet teacher opened up an exercise class in her neighborhood. That class gave Elsie more than just bodily exercise, it gave her stress relief, fun, friends, and fabulous deportment tuition from an amazing former dancer!

Elsie found her 'thing'. The thing that helped her cope with stress and loss and the daily drudge. I hope and pray that you will find your 'thing'. Just keep looking and don't resort to desperate measures, they tend to have desperate results.

ഇൽ

This book looks at three national leaders and four people from entertainment & the arts. That's because there is a lot of information available about these people. We can find out what they ate, what they weighed, their lifestyles, and their emotional problems. I chose to feature them because they stood out in their fields and struggled terribly with their weight.

I hope you enjoy reading this book and that, if you have weight or health issues, it will help you to understand them and find healthy ways to deal with them. The people I studied when researching this book all took drastic steps to lose weight. In doing so, most of them ruined their health and many of them died as a direct or indirect result. There were other people I could have included – such as Orson Welles – but who I left out because their stories were too similar to the stories of those I did use.

We live in an age of food abundance but not nutrient abundance. Many of us are actually chronically malnourished, even if we look well-padded and over-fed. The people in this book certainly were.

But we are fortunate to live in the information age, and we can learn from what they went through. We don't have to make the same mistakes.

Mia

Part 1

Big National Leaders

Henry VIII

You might want to cut back on the meat

The Metropolitan Museum of Art's Gallery 371 houses the field armor of King Henry VIII of England. It is believed to be the armor that he wore on his last military campaign, the siege of Boulogne in France in 1544-46.

He was aged 53 and near the end of his eventful life. His armor gives us an insight into his weight at that time. It is clear that he was really **very** big. When compared to armor that he wore when he was a young, athletic prince, we can see just how massively overweight he was.

In Tudor times, most people were shorter than they are now – you can tell by the beds and doorframes of the period. The average height for a man was 5' 6'. Henry was between 6' 1' and 6' 2' tall, which must have made him an impressive sight, especially when he was young and fit. It will surely have helped him gain the respect of the 'little people' around him – he must have towered over most of them quite considerably.

By the end of his reign, though, he was almost as wide as he was tall. We know this because quite detailed records were kept by the staff who looked after his clothing requirements. His last armor was built to make room for his 52' waist and 53' chest.

The Royal Armouries in London houses some armor he wore when he was in his 20s. His waist then was just 32' and his chest 39'. That's neat for such a tall guy.

When Henry was 24 he was described by an ambassador from Venice as:

> **'The handsomest potentate I ever set eyes on, with an extremely fine calf to his leg and a round face so very beautiful that it would become a pretty woman.'**
>
> (Pasqualigo, 1515)

So we can gather that he changed quite a bit over the course of his long and eventful life.

Why and how he changed is worth looking at, because it gives us big clues behind the reasons many people struggle with weight gain today. There were no fast-food restaurants to blame back in the Tudor period. No sodas or TV dinners. No factory foods. Yet they still had weight problems.

Let's take a look at Henry's life to see what went wrong for him.

Henry's Early Life

Henry wasn't born as heir to the throne of England. His older brother Arthur drew that short straw. That meant that Arthur was sent away at a tender age to a Welsh castle where his own household looked after him. He wasn't allowed to play rough or dangerous games, instead he was taught how to be a prince.

Henry wasn't as valuable so was left with his mother and sisters, where he experienced far more freedom and fun. He spent much of his childhood and early adulthood engaged in activity – jousting, riding, dancing, archery. It made him healthy and muscular. He was considered one of the best jousters in England, as well as a talented tennis player and wrestler.

The history books show that Henry had a number of quite serious sporting accidents. The first was a jousting accident in 1524 (when he was 33) and it left him with debilitating migraine-type headaches for the rest of his life. In 1527 he got a nasty foot injury while playing tennis.

It was to be a jousting accident which contributed to much of his later deterioration as it meant he could no longer take part in the sports he loved.

Henry's Eating Habits

When we look back at the Tudor period, we imagine that the wealthy people ate at banquets every night, tearing the meat off bones with their teeth. That is only partly true!

We know a fair bit about the eating habits of the Tudors from historical records. A dig into them is quite surprisingly. Far from being rough in their eating habits, wealthy Tudors seem to have had quite discerning palates.

Contrary to popular belief, fruit **was** eaten and it was occasionally eaten raw. I had read in my school history books that Tudors only ate cooked fruits – e.g. in pies – but I was delighted to discover that Henry enjoyed fresh cherries and strawberries. He even introduced apricots to Britain and had lots of apricot trees planted at one of his favorite palaces, Nonsuch. He may have been influenced in his fruit-eating by his first wife, Catherine of Aragon. Catherine was from Spain and would have grown up eating an abundance of fresh local foods.

Henry also seemed to enjoy vegetables, as he employed a gardener specially to grow salad vegetables for him.

He did have a sweet tooth, though (the healthy downfall of many people!). His kitchens housed confectioneries and pastry houses and even his red wine was very sweet. He didn't drink water – no-one did. They hydrated themselves with beer and ale and that very sweet red wine.

Expensive, rarer meats were the foods of kings and the aristocracy. Henry is known to have eaten thirteen dishes a day, many of them meat-based. He ate pork almost every day. Meat was eaten much less frequently by poorer people. The main staple of their diet was bread – generally a good, rough, homemade bread.

Richer folk could afford white bread, which they considered more of a delicacy – but actually it was less nutritious and more disease-provoking. Henry ate a lot of bread, all of it believed to be white.

Henry's Early Health

Henry inherited a good constitution from his father, Henry VII. Old Henry had won the English throne on the battlefield so we can assume he was fairly robust and healthy.

Henry VII had married Elizabeth of York, old King Edward IV's daughter. She was a good bet because her mother, Elizabeth Woodville (the 'White Queen') had been very fertile, producing ten children. In those days, childbirth was painful and dangerous, with many women dying either in childbirth or as a result of it soon afterwards. Not so Elizabeth Woodville, who remained hearty and healthy throughout, despite living under enormous stress. She helped arrange her daughter, Elizabeth's, marriage[2] to Henry Tudor, who became Henry VII.

So Henry came from good, healthy stock, which partly explained his ability to withstand the diseases – such as smallpox, plague, and sweating sickness – which were such a problem in Tudor England (it didn't help three of his six siblings, though, who died young).

---

[2] It was a good match in many ways as Elizabeth was a Plantagenet, the old dynasty. It helped heal the wounds of war and unite two dynasties.

He was healthier than his elder brother, Arthur, whose death (believed to be from the sweating sickness) made Henry the sudden heir to the throne.

One of the things that we know Henry suffered from was constipation. With all the white bread he ate, that's hardly surprising!

Henry's Later Health

If you ask someone what they know about Henry VIII, they will generally say that he had six wives and that he was very fat. Some people will also add that he had syphilis, the venereal disease. Actually, that's been disproven (Devonald, 1963[3]). The standard Tudor treatment for syphilis was with mercury (yes, really, the cure was more likely to kill than the illness!) but no record has been found of it being prescribed for Henry. As Henry kept very good records, we can fairly safely assume that if it wasn't recorded, it probably wasn't prescribed and he had no need of it.

He is widely suspected to have suffered from impotence. Anne Boleyn, his second wife, is known to have complained that Henry was sometimes unable to 'perform' sexually. This was an issue for her as she wanted to give Henry his longed-for son (and also give herself some security, he had dispensed with his first wife for being unable to give him a son). This does make sense as impotence is not uncommon in overweight men.

---

[3] http://journals.ed.ac.uk/resmedica/article/viewFile/403/684

Constipation began to be a huge problem for Henry and probably contributed to his obesity. He weighed nearly 400lbs in his later years.

A jousting accident – which happened while he was married to Anne Boleyn – was severe enough to knock him out for two hours. That's a pretty bad concussion. Some medical experts now believe that it actually caused brain damage and could partly explain his famous rages and bloodlust. Henry is known to have had thousands of people executed – perhaps up to 72,000. Two of them were his wives, Anne and her cousin Kathryn Howard. Anne's death came shortly after Henry's catastrophic accident.

He had a recurring open wound (probably a varicose ulcer) on his leg throughout his later life. It wasn't helped by the lack of medical knowledge at the time. His physicians would not let it heal, as they believed it was important to encourage the toxins to leave the body. So every time it started to close up, they would open it again to let the 'bad' out. It must have been extremely painful for Henry and would no doubt have caused depression.

What Went Wrong For Henry?

Henry had had almost inexhaustible energy in his youth. He came from very healthy parents, he survived horrendous illnesses that wiped out thousands of other people, and he had the best, most expensive foods available to him.

So why did he end up as a bloated, pain-ridden caricature of his former athletic self?

Briefly, it was due to his:

1. **Diet** - he are a *lot* of meat and bread.
2. **Reckless sports** - Henry was reputed to be fearless. He loved the thrill of the jousting arena, as well as the hunt. It was a jousting accident that probably caused his leg injury, which meant that he could no longer participate in sports at all.
3. **Inactivity** - in later years he became almost completely inactive, thanks to the pain in his leg.

The other thing we can't ignore is Henry's mental health. He was a witty, humorous youth but turned into a murderous bloated monster. What happened? Experts have several theories but two stand out.

GUILT

Henry – like many people of his time – was religious. Not only that, he was a Catholic (i.e. Roman Catholic). That may seem strange for the founder of the Church of England but he remained, in most ways, very Catholic.

He wanted to divorce Catherine and marry Anne Boleyn. The only way to get his divorce, as the Pope wouldn't grant it, was to break with Rome. That break didn't just involved Henry himself but his whole country.

All this happened around the time of Martin Luther and the blossoming of Protestantism so it was very timely.

People have since assumed that Henry became a Protestant but he didn't, he just found it convenient to set up his own church so he could get what he wanted – his divorce, a new wife, and the possibility of sons.

Henry plundered monasteries and had abbots and priests (as well as Protestant ministers) executed. Yet he remained Catholic in his beliefs. There would have been some guilt. Guilt can make a person go crazy and Henry certainly did appear to lose his marbles.

He was finally free from Catherine and her supporters in 1536, when she died from what we now know was cancer. There is debate over Henry's behavior at mass that day – and color of Anne's dress, she wore bright yellow - after receiving the news. Some Anne-favoring historians have explained this away as yellow being the color of mourning in Spain (Catherine was Spanish).

That doesn't seem to have been the case though. In *Manners, Customs & Observances*, author Leopold Wagner explains that both black and white are the colors of mourning throughout Europe and were during Henry VI's time – not yellow. He points out that prior to 1498:

> *'Anne, queen of Charles VIII of France, surrounded her coat of arms with black drapery and dessed herself in black on the death of her husband, in opposition to the prevailing custom, widows in England, France, and Spain generally adopted white mourning.'*

Wagner does mention that yellow is a mourning color in both Egypt and Burma and that in Brittany widows' caps are yellow. So perhaps Henry and Anne were just misinformed and/or bad at geography rather than callous!

Whether or not Henry was jubilant at the news of Catherine's death, he did show some emotion afterwards. He received a letter from her and sobbed when he read it.

Whatever he truly felt and believed, the whole incident was a very stressful time for him (and his people).

The same month, Henry's catastrophic jousting accident happened.

INJURY

The jousting accident that caused his dreadful leg injury perhaps caused more injuries than there appeared to be on the surface. What happened was that his horse fell on him. A big, heavy, unmovable animal landing on top of anyone is going to do a lot of damage.

Added to that was the fact that he was unconscious for around two hours. That is long enough to startle any emergency room physician today – for his doctors and attendants back then it must have been dreadful. It almost certainly did long-term damage to his brain.

Anne's fall from grace happened just months after this and added to Henry's mental problems.

He was never the same again. He became suspicious of

everyone's motives (rightly so in many cases) and paranoid. Gruesome executions – beheadings and burnings – increased. Anyone who disagreed with the king faced death and even those closest to him lived in fear of their lives. This was a far cry from the popular, happy prince Henry had been when his reign started.

What Can We Learn From Henry?

DON'T EAT A TUDOR-STYLE DIET[4]

The quantity of food rather than the quality seems to have been the big problem. Court culture was to eat a lot, around 13 dishes a day. They sometimes ate 10 portions of meat over just two courses.

Henry's diet was studied by the makers of the documentary *Inside the body of Henry VIII*. By reading court records, letters, and official papers, they guess that his regular caloric intake was 5,000 calories per day – twice the recommended intake for a man.[5]

Henry seems to have eaten even more meat than most rich Tudors, especially red meat, which he particularly enjoyed. He even had what he called 'flesh days' when he ate just meat (Atkins, anyone?!). That was particularly hard on his digestion and must have contributed to his problems with severe constipation, which started troubling him in middle age. (Lipscomb & Betteridge, 2013)

---

[4] https://suite.io/tracey-white/5qzy2nv
[5] http://youtu.be/fCbZ60q9NYo

Rich Tudors ate meat (generally roasted) at every meal and a lot of pork in particular. Pork is very prone to going rancid and some people believe that one of the reasons it was banned in the the Bible for the Israelites was for health reasons. Pigs can carry tapeworm, hepatitis E, and other parasites and viruses (Axe[6]).

Meat, if you choose to eat it, is best as a ***part*** of your diet, not a staple. The healthiest peoples in the world – and in history – are/were either vegetarian or did not include animal flesh as a large part of their diet.

GO EASY ON THE ALCOHOL

The Tudors didn't drink water as they lacked the technology to purify it. Drinking water was actually dangerous but turning it into ale (beer) made it safe, killing germs and parasites. So they drank a LOT of ale. Every time we would drink a glass of water today, they would drink ale.

Henry seems to have drunk more than most. His thirst was said to be unquenchable – another sign of a poor diet. (Lipscomb & Betteridge, 2013) He is said to have drunk 10 pints of beer per day, as well as a lot of [sweetened] red wine.

One of the reasons for his thirst was probably his excessive meat intake. Meat was salted in order to preserve it. His body would also have been crying out for water in order to detoxify.

---

[6]   http://draxe.com/why-you-should-avoid-pork/

DO HEALTHY EXERCISE, NOT RISKY SPORTS

From history books and court documents, we know that Henry was a very athletic prince. Those who knew him commented on his 'Superabundance of nervous energy' (Lipscomb & Betteridge, 2013).

Paolo da Lodi, the Milanese ambassador at court at the time commented:

> *'[Henry] is never still or quiet... He does wonders and leaps like a stag [at dancing].'*

That sounds like nervous energy – which he dealt with on the hunting field, at jousting tournaments, and via vigorous dancing. Once he could no longer get rid of his energy, he would have become frustrated and despondent.

The injuries he sustained on the jousting field could have been avoided if he had taken up less dangerous sports.

DON'T IGNORE DIABETES

Medical historians now believe that Henry suffered from undiagnosed diabetes. There's probably not much his doctors could have done to manage it back then but there is a lot we can do now.

Unmanaged diabetes is potentially deadly. It increases the risk of getting other complaints too, illnesses such as: foot and leg pain (even amputation – which Henry's doctors wouldn't have dared to suggest), nerve damage, skin problems, high blood pressure, kidney disease, eye problems, and heart disease.

Diets low in fat and sugar are best to both prevent and control diabetes. The actress Halle Berry was diagnosed with Type 2 diabetes after she collapsed on the set of a TV show. She was in a coma for a week and could have died. In an interview[7] with the UK's Daily Mail newspaper she said that her doctors told her what unmanaged diabetes could do:

> *'They told me I might lose my eyesight, or I could lose my legs ... They explained that, due to excess sugar in the body, diabetics can suffer kidney failure, have a five times higher risk of developing heart disease, and 80% of people with diabetes will die from cardiovascular complications.'*

Scary stuff. But totally manageable nowadays, thanks to improved knowledge about diet, as well as excellent drugs that can control insulin when diet alone isn't enough. Halle completely overhauled her diet. She now eats a diet low in fat, sugar, and processed carbohydrates. She also took the advice of a personal trainer as she understood that stress affects blood sugar and exercise helps it.

---

[7] http://www.dailymail.co.uk/health/article-371528/Halle-Berry-My-battle-diabetes.html

DON'T GIVE UP AN ACTIVE LIFESTYLE

Henry stopped his athletic activities after his jousting accident. The lack of movement meant his blood circulation will have slowed, oxygen transportation would have been inefficient and the result was that his leg never actually healed.

Lack of mobility causes weight gain if you keep eating the same as you did when you were more active and in Henry's case the weight gain was colossal. Most of us know the feeling of resorting to food to 'cure' a psychological pain. Henry would no doubt have felt frustrated at being so inactive and depressed by the pain he was in, the smell that came from his suppurating leg ulcer, and the never-ending weight gain. He had been a handsome, athletic prince, turning into a bloated ogre must have been agony for him – and his ego.

We are fortunate in the 21st century to have machines and methods that we can use to make up in some way for lack of ability to take part in exercise and active hobbies.

$$\text{\textbf{ÕÕÕ}}$$

Let's turn to another big historical figure, a monarch again, who was born just over 100 years after Henry but suffered a similar fate…

Queen Anne of England

One of the first chocoholics

Queen Anne was the name of Henry VIII's short-lived second wife, Anne Boleyn. Her namesake, who reigned in her own right a century later, isn't as well known and isn't even one of the most famous British monarchs but I have featured her here because her weight was significant and well-documented.

Queen Anne is best remembered in, of all things, furniture! 'Queen Anne legs' are a feature of both antiques and some modern furniture. She wasn't known personally for her legs – she lived in a time of long dresses and horror of showing even an ankle. The leg thing came about because furniture during her reign had a particular look.

Anne was born in 1665 - just over a century after King Henry VIII died - into an entirely different dynasty. King Henry's youngest daughter, Elizabeth (who, interestingly, didn't have weight problems), was the last of the Tudors, dying in 1603. The next dynasty was the Stuarts, starting with Mary, Queen of Scots' son James I[8], and ending with Anne, as she didn't have any surviving children.

Anne's grandfather, Charles I, was James I's son. Charles had been the first (and only) English monarch to be executed by the government. His sons, Charles (later Charles II) and James (later James II), had managed to escape to mainland Europe – in the case of James, by dressing as a girl! Because of this, and continuing political and religious upheaval, Anne grew up in a climate of fear.

Charles II, Anne's uncle, was the reigning king when she was born. Charles had been able to return after England struggled through a disastrous decade as a republic and almost descended into anarchy after the death of the parliamentary leader, Oliver Cromwell.

This tumultuous period was just after the time of the Pilgrims, who had left England because of the rules James I brought in, which prevented their religious freedom. The Puritans, as one branch of the Pilgrims became, had left because they wanted to 'purify' the English church – the Church of England – of Roman Catholic influences. But Anne's father (Charles II's brother), was Catholic. Tension in their Church of England (aka Protestant) family was high. It didn't help Anne that her mother died when the little girl was just 6 years old. Her father remarried and her new stepmother was just six years older than her!

---

[8]   James was actually James I of England and VI of Scotland!

Even later on when Anne's sister became Queen, the tensions remained. Queen Mary feared Anne's popularity and fertility – Mary was unable to produce children. Hostilities were barely beneath the surface between the two sisters and this will have had a profound effect on Anne's mental health. She was reported as being 'morose'.

One good thing was Anne's marriage to Prince George of Denmark. They seem to have been happy together, at least initially. In later life George took to drinking and became a bit of a bore!

Anne's Reproductive Problems

Lots of queens suffered the heartbreak of multiple miscarriages and stillbirths. King Henry VIII's first and second wives were both afflicted. Queen Anne, over a century later, endured the same problem. She was particularly unfortunate, as only one of her [probably] 18[9] pregnancies resulted in a live birth. Then that son, William, died at the age of 11.

So we know that Queen Anne was very fertile, which was a sign of good health. It isn't clear why she was unable to produce live babies though. In his book *Queen Anne* Edward Gregg reports that one of her stillbirths was said to be due to a fall from a horse, which is entirely plausible. Medical records of her other miscarriages and stillbirths don't shed any light

---

[9] Historians can't agree on the number of Anne's pregnancies. It varies between 17 and 19, according to who you read!

on other likely causes though.

We do know that the possibly 20 years that she was pregnant or in some stage of pregnancy took a great toll on her health. Many of her pregnancies took place during times of massive change.

Anne's Declining Health

Anne didn't get a great start in life, health-wise. She was a sickly child and contracted smallpox when she was 12. She also had poor vision and problems with her eyes, and is believed to have had porphyria, an inherited blood disease.

Her health deteriorated more once her many miscarriages and stillbirths got underway. In fact, one court official reported that she wasn't expected to live very long (Gregg, 2001) and she suffered prolonged illnesses following several of the pregnancies.

Her sister Mary was expected to outlive her, as many believed Anne's failing health would result in her becoming an invalid and suffering an early death.

Anne wasn't without some defenses, though. Her sister died young as a result of smallpox – but Anne was immune as she had already had it. She was pregnant again, of course, at this time!

Like many people who struggle with their health, Anne lost confidence in her doctors, and found new ones. She also tried going to the popular spa towns of Bath and Tunbridge Wells, which were renowned for their healing waters. Whether all this helped is open to question but she did live longer than expected so perhaps the doctors and spa treatments did some good.

Anne suffered badly from rheumatism. There are reports of her having to be carried outside if she wanted some air, and by the time she was 30 could no longer manage stairs. She also had some weakness in her legs which prevented her from standing properly.

Scholars have suggested that her eye problem – whatever it was – may have been the reason that she wasn't highly educated. As she wasn't expected to become queen, she wasn't educated as a first-born prince might have been. Lack of education will have affected her confidence and contributed to her later [alleged] drinking problems.

Her eye problem was severe enough for her to be sent abroad for treatment when she was little. Anne spent a year in France and came back 'very much improved both in her constitution and personal accomplishments.' (Somerset, 2013)

She seemed to be much better for a while but within a few years was 'ill of her eyes again' and her vision was to continue to be a problem. One of the people she consulted prescribed beer for this problem – to hydrate the brain, apparently! The eye problem left her with a slight squint, which caused her to look like she was frowning.

Apart from her physical health problems, she seems to have had another issue which could have resulted in difficulties. She displayed some bitterness towards her stepmother when she gave birth to a healthy child. Anne referred to the baby as 'it' and, after a token visit, didn't go back to see mother or child. That kind of bitterness can have physical effects.

Meanwhile, Anne's sad, unsuccessful pregnancies continued. She was reported to have been 'monstrously swollen' during one of her pregnancies, so much that her attendants thought it was illness rather than pregnancy. That one did result in a live birth, although the baby died soon after.

She started to show symptoms of depression and believed that her life would be cut short. In a letter to a friend, she said:

> *'I hope in the next world I shall be at ease but in this I find I must not expect it long together.'*

She was an invalid by the time she was just 35.

A servant of Anne's surviving son wrote a book about his experiences at the royal court. In *Memoirs of Prince William Henry, Duke of Gloucester* (Lewis, 1789), the little prince is portrayed as a sickly child with an anxious mother. Anne referred to him as 'my poor boy' and with good reason – he could barely walk until he was 5.

She was dreadfully worried about her son. When he suffered his final illness – smallpox – Anne spent every minute with him, sleeping next to his bed and fainting at one point.

Although she was only 37 when she took the throne, Anne was suffering dreadfully with gout and was unable to stand or walk at her own coronation. She was so overweight that her attendants had trouble finding ceremonial robes that would fit her for her first speech to Parliament. At her funeral, her coffin was noticably large and required 14 men to carry it.

One of the contributing factors to her gout problem will no doubt have been her addiction to brandy. She was known popularly as 'Brandy Nan'. She kept brandy in a little teapot and helped herself to it regularly.

She may even have been prescribed brandy. In the 1700s, doctors didn't know that alcohol in general and spirits in particular made gout worse. A book written in the following century even had recipes containing brandy that were supposed to help gout! (*Food for the Invalid*, Fothergill, 1880)

We now know, of course, that alcohol is disastrous for gout sufferers. Victor Konshin in *Beating Gout: A Sufferer's Guide to Living Pain Free* says:

> *Drinking alcohol is one of the most significant lifestyle factors affecting gout. Alcohol causes both an increase in the production of uric acid as well as a decrease in excretion. It is also a diuretic (which causes the body to lose water), further increasing the concentration of uric acid in the body.*

Yet it is understandable to want an alcoholic drink when you are in pain. It 'takes the edge off', numbs the feelings a little, and gives the world a slightly hazy appearance that is preferable to reality.

About That Leg Thing

Furniture with ball and claw feet became popular during Anne's reign. It was the start of furniture being thought of as more than just something to sit on – it had to be something pretty to look at as well.

There is no connection with Queen Anne legs on furniture and the queen's health problems with her legs. That's just a coincidence – but it helps history students remember a few facts!

The fact that furniture became something more than just practical was an indication that things were picking up for the country during Anne's reign. Life wasn't so hard anymore, people were able to invest in things they enjoyed rather than just things to help them survive.

There were some brilliant military victories during her time on the throne – including the British capture of Gibraltar and the battle of Blenheim. The UK was actually created at this time, when England and Scotland were unified. Now Anne was queen of the United Kingdom of Great Britain. Her reign paved the way for another golden age.

Anne's Death

Anne died, after a short reign, in 1714. The official cause of death was stroke but experts at the time said it was due to erysipelas and suppressed gout.

Erysipelas is a nasty rash – sometimes known as St Anthony's fire. It causes fever, fatigue, headache, vomiting, swollen lymph glands, shaking, chills, and chronic swelling of the extremities.

It is now known to be caused by – mostly – a streptococci bacteria which can enter the skin via insect bites, eczema, scratches, athlete's foot, ulcers, or even via the nasal passages.

It is common in the elderly, young children, people with immune deficiency, diabetes, alcoholism, fungal infections, and lymphatic drainage problems.

Nowadays, it can be treated with antibiotics but if it is allowed to continue without treatment it can spread to deeper tissue and cause necrotizing fasciitis – the flesh-eating bug. It is known to have caused the death of the baseball player/manager Miller Huggins, who managed the Yankees from 1918-1929 – Babe Ruth and Lou Gehrig's time.

What Went Wrong For Anne?

In her youth, Anne had enjoyed dancing but had to give it up once her mobility problems set in (Winn, 2014). This follows the pattern set by King Henry VIII, who gave up his athletic activities following his jousting accident and then piled weight on.

If Anne had been able to take up some other sort of movement that she could manage, it could have prevented much of her later obesity and further deterioration. If she was alive today there would be plenty of options available to her: swimming, Pilates, yoga, massage, passive exercise machines. In her era, though, people just didn't understand that movement is life.

Other things we know that Anne suffered from she could well have made worse by her eating and drinking habits:

> Miscarriages and stillbirths

> A problem with her eyes

> Gout

> Rheumatism

> Porphyria

That's quite a load! Porphyria in particular is very interesting. It is believed to be the illness that inspired the vampire phenomenon. An article on the website, Power Of The Gene[10], claims that Bram Stoker, the author of *Dracula*, met a patient who had the symptoms of porphyria – which include photosensitivity and a dislike of being in the sun.

If Anne had porphyria, it was probably from her family

---

[10]   http://powerofthegene.com/joomla/index.php/conversational-genetics/genetics-in-legends-and-folklaw

line. Mary Queen of Scots, her son James I, and James's son Henry all suffered from the disease. It is possible that Anne inherited it too.

Porphyria can cause abdominal pain and constipation so perhaps it had something to do with Anne's difficulties with reproduction and love of brandy – as brandy would have numbed the pain.

Anne's love of chocolate seems to have been the biggest cause of her weight gain – accompanied by her inability to exercise due to gout and leg pain. In *Queen Anne: Patroness of Arts* (Winn, 2014), the author quotes someone who knew the family:

> *'Her body growing extremely fat and unwieldy, she disused hunting and other diversions that might have been conducive to her health, and which, perhaps, might have been longer preserved if she had not eat so much, an unhappiness derived to her ex traduce, not from her father, who was abstemious enough, but from her mother; and not supped so much chocolate: I say, she was grown monstrously fat.'*

Royals could afford to eat and drink to excess and the Stuarts certainly did – they 'believed excess to be a sign of royalty' (Winn, 2014). Anne's mother is known to have had a great love of eating, so perhaps it was natural that Anne herself would lean towards excess.

Her constant self-medicating with brandy could well

have contributed to her reproductive problems. The UCSF Medical Center states that:

> *'Drinking alcohol can increase the risk of miscarriage, stillbirth, newborn death, and fetal alcohol syndrome.'*[11]

If Anne was a big drinker she was going slightly away from the norm as the Stuart era saw the start of coffee and chocolate houses. The drinking of beer declined as more people drank coffee, tea, and hot chocolate. (Kings and Queens - The Stuarts - 1603-1714)

Perhaps that is why chocolate was one of Anne's downfalls. Like her mother before her, she liked to drink her chocolate. Drinking our calories is always a bad idea, we can take in far more than we realize.

What Can We Learn From Anne?

WE NEED TO LEARN A BETTER RESPONSE TO STRESS

You can't control the level of stress you are under but you can control your reaction to it. Stress does indeed kill and it seems our brains know this and come up with all sorts of tricks to help us. But those tricks can kill us.

Comfort eating generally involves large quantities of

---

[11] http://www.ucsfhealth.org/education/substance_use_during_pregnancy/

refined carbohydrates. We know that carbs cause a change in the brain that is similar to the change that taking heroin causes.

Dr David Ludwig is a Professor of Nutrition at the Boston Children's Hospital. He investigates the reasons for obesity. One of his many studies looked at how food affects the dopamine regions of the brain. Dopamine is a hormone that functions as a neurotransmitter in the brain. It has many functions but some very relevant ones both for those who want to lose weight and people who live with chronic pain.

➢ Decreased dopamine levels are associated with higher pain – dopamine acts like an analgesic.

➢ Some antidepressant medications act on dopamine pathways – indicating dopamine's effects on mood.

➢ Dopamine acts on the prefrontal cortex of the brain, affecting how we respond to things.

➢ Dopamine is released in the brain in response to experiences that the brain decides are rewarding.

So dopamine is great and we need to find ways of boosting it naturally. Dopamine is boosted by eating foods that are rich in tyrosine. Good sources of tyrosine include:

➢ Almonds

➢ Peanuts (which could be why many of us have trouble stopping eating peanuts! Tim Ferriss, author of The Four-Hour Body says he notices that, *'Peanut butter is like crack cocaine for some women - for whom a tablespoon of peanut butter means trying to balance the entire contents of a jar on a spoon!')*

➢ Sesame seeds
➢ Pumpkin seeds
➢ Bananas
➢ Watermelons
➢ Spirulina
➢ Blueberries
➢ Turkey

Other things we can do to increase dopamine levels are:

➢ Exercise
➢ Deep breathing
➢ Relaxing activities
➢ Avoiding processed foods – especially those high in fat and sugar

KEEP ACTIVE – WHATEVER IT TAKES

We are so fortunate now. We don't have to give up all movement if we become unable to exercise. There are machines that can move our limbs for us, massage therapists to keep our circulation and lymph healthy, and – if budget is an issue - free health habits we can take up that help tremendously, such as dry skin brushing.[12]

---

[12] http://amzn.com/0992960908 (Shameless plug - I wrote a book on

TAKE UP HOBBIES THAT DON'T REQUIRE SITTING DOWN

Anne was known to be a fan of cards. Card games are usually played while eating and drinking. Try to find hobbies that don't involve lots of physical inactivity and social eating/drinking – that's a bad combination!

EAT WELL

Anne doesn't appear to have eaten healthily. That could well have had a bearing on her reproductive problems. The same thing, from a different angle, happened to King Henry VIII's first wife, Catherine of Aragon. Catherine too only managed to produce one child who survived infancy. She had many miscarriages and stillbirths. It was a cause of great heartbreak to her and eventually led to her divorce as the king desperately wanted a son to follow him – he got rid of Catherine in favor of Anne Boleyn.

Catherine, in desperation for a son, turned to her faith. She was a devoted, pious woman and a faithful Roman Catholic. She did a lot of fasting and praying in the hope that her piety would persuade God to give her a son.

However, even the Pope realized that women need to eat in order to get pregnant and produce healthy children. He wrote to say that he thought she may be over-doing the fasting! One of the Spanish ambassadors also wrote that:

---

dry skin brushing – but only because it gives such amazing, quick results!)

> *'Irregularity in her eating makes her unwell. Which is why she does not menstruate well.'*

With low calorie and strict detox diets being so popular in our era, we would do well to remember Catherine's sad experience.

DON'T DRINK YOUR CALORIES

Hot chocolate is delicious but packed with calories. If you enjoy chocolate, a few small squares of dark chocolate will give you the 'hit' you need without a huge amount of fat.

Even healthy drinks such as fruit juices and smoothies can be a problem if you need to lose weight, or don't want to put any on. Eating whole fruit instead of its juice is an important first step. You could drink the juice of 8 oranges but probably not be able to eat 8 full oranges!

Smoothies can be a healthy choice if you make them yourself (and add dopamine-boosting seeds). Store-bought smoothies are often packed with cheaper ingredients and use processed fruit juice. They also don't tend to include things that can make you full such as seeds and oats. Put those in your own smoothie and it will keep you full for hours.

BE CAREFUL WITH ALCOHOL

Alcohol almost certainly made Anne's gout worse. If you don't have gout, don't encourage it by over-doing the alcohol. It dehydrates, depletes vitamins and minerals, affects mood, and – ultimately – can cause brain damage.

ॐ

We think of comfort/stress eating as a modern thing but there was a US President who became very large mainly due to being unhappy. We'll look at him next…

President William Howard Taft

Unhappiness can be life-threatening

Ask a non-American to name a US president and I'll bet you a big bag of fudge that none of them think of Taft. In fact, ask dozens of Americans to name 10 US presidents and I seriously doubt the poor old 27th would make the lists of more than about 1% of them.

He was the second president of the 20th century, coming after Theodore Roosevelt and before Woodrow Wilson. Those two towering figures still overshadow Taft a century later. Other presidents are remembered for great events or decisions: Lincoln for making the Thanksgiving tradition official; Wilson for establishing Mother's Day. Task gave us Tax Day and the Oval Office, among other things, but he is only known for his massive girth.

When I started researching obesity through the ages, Taft came up as an obese president and I half-heartedly looked him up – then got hooked and started devouring all the information I could find about him. I felt sorry for him, more than anything else: he was an intelligent, caring man who is almost forgotten by history. This despite being the only person to have served as both President and Chief Justice – you would think people would remember that!

Taft's Early Life & Health

The man who would later be known as 'Big Lub' at Yale was born in 1857 into a powerful political family. He was heavy from the day he was born. When he was seven weeks old, his mother wrote:

> *'He is very large of his age and grows fat every day... He has such a large waist, that he cannot wear any of the dresses that are made with belts.'*
>
> Pringle, 1986

He grew into a tall (5' 11.5'), attractive, and jolly boy but always had quite a heavy build – even though he was as active as other children of the period. One of his schools required a mile-long walk up a steep hill every day and there are no reports that he struggled with it.

At the age of nine, he was in an accident in his family carriage when the horses ran unexpectedly. He suffered from a slight skull fracture and a bad cut on the head. This caused what observers called a 'deep depression' in his skull that remained throughout his life. (Health & Medical History of President William Taft, 2000-2013)

He wasn't a big drinker, even at college and went teetotal a few years before becoming President.

Taft's Weight Problems

When Taft graduated from Yale he weighed 243lbs – but most people thought he carried it well. By the time he was 48, though, he had ballooned to 320lbs.

What happened? The main reason seems to be that he went into politics – and didn't want to.

His weight fluctuated wildly over the years, as he sought the advice of doctors. Under English physician Dr. N. E. Yorke-Davies, he lost 70lbs over the course of a year and a half. But he put almost all of it back on, rising to over 300lbs again.

At the end of his presidency he weighed 335-340lbs before going down to 270lbs in just over a year. Going on body mass index – which can safely do as he wasn't a heavily-muscled athlete – he was severely obese even at 240lbs.

Given his obesity, there has been speculation over the years that the head injury he got at the age of 9 when the family's horses ran off damaged his pituitary gland, which caused his obesity.

It is understandable that people would think that – it has been given as a possible reason the biblical figure Goliath was so tall (Bear, Conners, & Paradiso, 2007).

In Taft's case it is unlikely - or at least a coincidence. We know that Taft was big from birth so his weight problems started very early on. Also, throughout his life, his weight fluctuated with his levels of stress and unhappiness. He was a classic comfort eater.

Although he did well at school, his parents were concerned that he was lazy and that:

> **'The high grades he earned came [only] as a result of their prodding.'**
>
> Lurie, 2012

So said parents through the ages!

Their prodding may have done some damage to Taft's self-esteem. Some writers have noted that he seemed to have a lifelong need for other people to urge him on – firstly his parents and brothers, and later his wife. Whether or not his parents withheld love and affection when Taft didn't perform as they wanted is open to speculation. If they did, it could go some way to explaining his later comfort eating.

Taft's ancestors dated back to the Massachusetts Bay Colony and many of them went into law. Taft's father also went into law and made Attorney General before becoming an ambassador. This heritage made Taft's progress through school and college swift. His father went to Yale and studied law, so did his brothers – he didn't have much choice.

His parents are described in one biography as 'devoted

but demanding' (Lurie, 2012). His father was a man of his era, quite proper and austere. His children saw a different side to him though. When his boys were away, Taft senior didn't like it, finding it too quiet:

> *'There is no noise and no mischief ... and on the whole it is not satisfactory to have no mischief about the house.'*

When Taft junior reached Yale he joined the Skull & Bones undergraduate secret society. (A fictional member of the Skull & Bones is Montgomery Burns of *The Simpsons*.)

Skull & Bones members are called 'Bonesmen' and Bonesmen do very well for themselves.[13] They employ and promote other Bonesmen and give all kinds of assistance to them – privately, professionally, and politically. Bonesmen hold positions of power; Taft employed two of them in his cabinet. The Tafts can count nine members of their family who have been Bonesmen.

After Yale, Taft went to law school but found it tedious so took a part-time job as a reporter for a local newspaper. He also spent time at his father's law office, which suited him much better than the dry classes at law school.

He said his time at the law office:

---

[13] Members of the Bush family have done rather well from their connections with the Bonesmen too!

> *'Has the effect of making me absorb some
> of the practical workings of the law.'*

Perhaps he was a kinesthetic learner, who needed to move and do in order to learn and understand information.

What Went Wrong For Taft

Taft went into politics (it was a Bonesmen tradition, after all) and became President Theodore Roosevelt's War Secretary before winning the Republican party presidential nomination. Why he allowed himself to be talked into running for the presidency is a mystery because he didn't seem to want to do it. His wife, brother, and Roosevelt himself managed to convince him. Roosevelt hand-selected Taft as his successor.

Taft, however, hated the campaign trail, saying it was:

> *'The most uncomfortable
> four months of my life.'*

The top job didn't make him big but it did make him bigger. He ballooned to 344lbs within a year. His nickname from the press quickly became 'Big Bill' and that was just the start of the fat jokes. He was depicted in cartoons as items of food and was given gifts of massive pieces of food by well-meaning fans and visitors.

While he took this all well – fulfilling the jolly fat person caricature perfectly – he was terribly unhappy during this period. As many people today understand, eating 'junk' food (generally fast-releasing, highly processed carbohydrates such as sugar and baked goods – the foods that Taft loved) can bring on a feeling of relaxation and slightly euphoria. It's similar to the feeling that strong drugs give and it is very addictive. Taft numbed his feelings with food – and it had a big effect.

Ask anyone who manages to remember Taft at all and they will probably mention the time when he allegedly got stuck in a bath tub and needed help getting out. Did it happen? We don't really know. There is a lot of rumor and not much evidence.

One mention of Taft and a bath tub is in The National Archive. There is a letter from the captain of a ship that Taft was due to travel on. The captain ordered a new, extra long and strong bed and mattress and an extra-wide bath tub for the President's cabin. There is no official mention of him getting stuck in that tub. The press reported that it was big enough to house 'four ordinary men'. If it was that big, it is unlikely that he managed to get stuck in it.

A book by Ike Hoover, a White House usher during Taft's presidency, does mention him getting stuck in a bath tub in the White House. However, the book was published in 1932 – almost 20 years after Taft left the presidency.

If it did happen, it seems odd that there is no other

official record of the event.

Taft's Health Problems

Taft was known for falling asleep at public events and companions commented on him not being alert after meals.

More seriously, he was also spotted panting for breath when walking, a sign that his obesity was having more long-term effects. He almost fainted while playing golf – possibly his first recorded manifestation of atrial fibrillation (abnormal heartbeat).

He is documented to have had other health problems that commonly plague those with weight problems, particularly high blood pressure, chronic indigestion and sleep apnea. The sleep apnea caused chronic, overwhelming tiredness due to lack of sleep. He was always tired – both mentally and physically.

Happily, he started on the road to improved health after losing the 1912 election. People as severely obese as he was often die young but Taft lived to the age of 72.

He lost a total of 70lbs and his sleep apnea in his first year as a former president and kept it off for the remainder of his life. Several years later he was appointed Chief Justice by his successor, Warren Harding but he had no more need for comfort eating. He was reported to be alert and attentive on the bench and ran the court well. The job must have suited him far more than politics - he stayed in it until just before his death in 1930.

By the time he was in his sixties, though, he was once again suffering from health problems. These were most likely caused by his earlier over-eating. He had an elevator fitted in his home, due to increasing immobility.

He died of heart disease, brought on by hardening of the arteries.

What Can We Learn From Taft?

Quite a lot according to Dr. Deborah Levine, a medical historian at Providence College in Rhode Island. She believes that Taft's experience of obesity:

> *'Sheds a lot of light on what we are going through now.'*

Dr Levine means the national obesity crisis. She believes today's obesity problems are the result of our increasingly sedentary lifestyles and the prevalence of fast foods.

Specifically, we can learn from Taft:

DON'T OVEREAT – ESPECIALLY MEAT

Taft was known for loving salmon and salads. These are modern super foods and not at all suspicious contributors to his massive weight.

It seems that it was the quantity of food he ate, rather than the quality, that was the problem. We know that

Mrs Taft appointed a dietician for her husband, as she was concerned about the amount he ate. He was concerned himself, commenting that:

> *'No real gentleman weighs more than 300lbs.'*

He seems to have had the comfort eater's attachment to food and fear of it not being available. He instructed that any trains he traveled on always had to have a well stocked dining car. He even specified that filet mignon[14] be available on his train journeys. He also enjoyed fish, turkey, and pork – having a combination of these at each regular lunch and dinner at the White House.

So we know that he particularly enjoyed meat products but there was something else that no doubt contributed to his weight problems. He loved baked things. Anything baked! His roast meals always included Yorkshire 'pudding', his lunches bread rolls, his breakfast waffles. Talk about carb overload!

He also frequently ordered sweet carbs: plum pudding, butterscotch cream pie, tapioca, steamed puddings, and fruit & cream tarts. His love of dairy products was encouraged by the gift of a milking cow from the Wisconsin Senator. The cow grazed on the front lawn of the Old Executive Office building.

He attributed his 70lb weight loss after leaving the presidency to cutting out bread, as well as pork and

---

[14] Beef steak

other fatty meats and fish. He also avoided alcohol and tobacco. He wrote, of this time in his life:

> *'I can truthfully say that I never felt any younger in all my life. Too much flesh is bad for any man.'*

He added that he ate a lot of all vegetables except potatoes. Modern commentators have likened his successful diet to the Atkins but it was nothing like it. While the Atkins emphasizes meat, Taft's diet minimized it and emphasized vegetables. It wasn't low carbohydrate – it was low **concentrated** carbohydrate.

DON'T LET OTHERS PERSUADE YOU TO DO SOMETHING YOU HATE

It looks like he found being President an overwhelming and stressful role and – more importantly – one that he never wanted. Many biographers (of both him and his wife) believe that he only took on the job to please his wife and improve his marriage.

That kind of self-sacrifice has an effect. The downtrodden wife and mother who swigs more sherry than she puts in the trifle and internalizes her anger rather than risk destabilizing the emotional climate in the home has more in common with a former president than she would ever imagine.

Apart from the effect on himself, there was another problem with him doing a job he didn't want. He wasn't very good at it. He is widely considered to have been a poor politician, much preferring law to politics.

If you allow others to persuade you to do something you don't want to do, it is extremely likely that you won't give it your heart and soul, that you aren't naturally skilled at it, and that you won't find it easy to learn how to get better at it. It's far better – for you and those around you - to do what you really want to do.

Taft managed to let go of the stress he suffered as President and felt that the office of Chief Justice was his greatest honor. He even wrote that he didn't remember that he was President. That's impressive. Being able to move on from our perceived failures and big stressors is important. They don't have to drag us down forever.

SUGAR EQUALS WEIGHT GAIN

Dr. Nathaniel Yorke-Davis, one of Taft's weight-loss physicians, wrote to him saying that on his recommended diet:

> *'Sugar is entirely debarred.'*

The doctor advised Taft to use saccharin, if he must, to sweeten foods – advice that wouldn't be given by any health-oriented doctors today. The dangers of saccharin weren't known then, clearly.

Modern weight-loss research agrees with the doctor's advice to avoid sugar though. Sugar has no nutritional value but that isn't the only reason it is bad news for dieters.

According to Dr Abram Hoffer, sugar causes cravings and addiction:

> *'Sugar is an addiction far stronger than what we see with heroin. It is the basic addictive substance from which all other addictions flow. Refined sugar and all refined foods such as polished rice, white flour and the like, are nothing less than legalized poisons.'*

FOOD QUANTITY MATTERS

Taft age huge portions – almost Henry VIII-sized portions. Tudors had an excuse for eating lots of calories. They lived active, often outdoor lives, in cold castles and houses. They needed more calories than we do today. The White House isn't exactly an igloo – whatever disillusioned tourists think about its size!

My ex-husband used to keep birds of prey. They were magnificent creatures that had tremendous power and massive wings. Yet they rarely flew voluntarily. We discovered that birds of prey don't fly for fun, only for food-finding purposes. It's because their food isn't high calorie and they easily burn through their available calories when flying, which uses up a tremendous amount of available energy. When flying, they would take any opportunity not to flap their wings, resting and letting thermals propel them. The problem with that was that the thermals could carry them many miles from home!

Today, many of us act like birds of prey. We seem to be scared that we will run out of calories in the midst of our daily lives and not be able to get home. But we usually have plenty of calories stored handily in our bodies, ready for conversion back into available energy.

We don't need massive quantities of food. We get the enjoyment of eating from small amounts – we often stop enjoying and tasting foods after the first couple of mouthfuls anyway.

Taft kept a food diary, which helped him, and that's still a good idea today. Paper and pen works, as do apps. MyFitnessPal is a great free app for mobile devices and desktop computers. It allows you to monitor your food intake and nutrition needs, as well as your weight and measurements. It can make a big difference.

⁝

National leaders are bound to be under massive amounts of stress - fending off wars and being forced to be diplomatic when they'd rather wring people by the neck! So let's take a look at some of the most privileged people on the planet, modern celebrities...

Part 2

Big People from Entertainment & The Arts

Alfred Hitchcock

Binging usually equals self-loathing

Alfred Hitchcock glares down his nose in many of his photos, dark eyes glaring and lips in a slight sneer. That snooty look wasn't actually snootiness, it was part of his armor – that and the suit of fat that he wore. The master of suspense was also a master of self-loathing.

Hitch's Early Life

Hitchcock was born right at the end of the 19th century, in 1899. His parents ran a wholesale grocery business in London and the family lived above the shop. A good early exposure to healthy fruits and vegetables didn't seem to help him later.

Young Alfred was a solitary chap, preferring studying maps and memorizing train schedules to playing with other children. He enjoyed trips with his parents though: with his father on produce-buying trips; and with both parents to plays and shows at the theatre. Those theatre trips were to make a lifelong impression on him.

He started his difficulties with food at an early age, binging in secret on things such as fried fish or bacon. His self-loathing also started then, as he was appalled at his over-eating and started another lifelong habit – crash dieting. (Wilson, 2013)

A story in *Alfred Hitchcock: Filming Our Fears* (Adair, 2002) shows the first instance that may have had a deep psychological effect on Alfred. When he was about 5 his father sent him, with a note, to the local police station as punishment for something he had done. The note obviously told the police sergeant to lock him in a cell for a few minutes, which the man did. Alfred later said that the incident gave him a 'lifelong terror of the police'. The book's author notes that many of the suspense films Alfred later made featured characters who had been falsely accused of crimes and were chased by authorities.

Alfred's fear of authority increased when he was sent to a Jesuit-run school that was famous for strict discipline and corporal punishment. Despite that, he did well at school, excelling in several subjects. He later said of his time there:

> *'The Jesuits taught me organization, control, and, to some degree, analysis. Their education is very strict, and orderliness is one of the things that came out of that.'*

Alfred's college education (he was studying to be an engineer) was cut short when his father died and he had to work to support himself and his mother. He took a job as a clerk at a telegraph company. He said the work was boring, which made him procrastinate as he didn't enjoy it. Like most procrastinators, he relied on the adrenaline rush when deadlines were looming to get him through.

He started taking evening classes and some of them were to prove very useful for his future in film-making: art history and drawing. His employers noticed his skill at drawing and transferred him to their advertising department. He started doing illustrations for the company magazine and even wrote stories for it. The magazine's first issue featured a dark tale of his that had echoes of his future films – suspense, terror, a twist in the tale. He signed the story 'Hitch'.

Hitch was a teenager when World War I started but he was too young initially and, when he became old enough, he failed the medical examination. This is the first indication we have of a health problem. Historians haven't unearthed what his health problem was but speculate that even then he could have been heavy and his weight would have been an issue for the army.

He still enjoyed going to plays and started going to the new movie theatres that were springing up in London – especially as movie tickets were cheaper than theatre tickets!

Hitch loved the movies so much that he started to read film journals – trade magazines that talked about the mechanics of film-making. It was one of those magazines that was to change his life. He read that a new film studio (a branch of an American company – Famous Players-Lasky) was opening in London. He hoped to land a job with the studio, using his drawing skills. He sketched some things that he thought might interest the studio, having read what their first production was going to be. After a false start – the studio scrapped their original plans and Hitch had to do more sketches – he was given a part-time job. For a while he juggled both jobs, until the studio took him on full-time just after he turned 21.

The studio gave him the perfect opportunity to study film-making first-hand. As a small operation, there wasn't a large staff and Hitch 'found himself doing a bit of everything'. (Adair, 2002)

When Anthony Hopkins played Hitch in *Hitchcock*, the 2012 film, his transformation into the famous director took a team of special effects people. Hopkins is slim and athletic himself and had to wear a big fatsuit and lots of facial prosthetics to take him up to Hitch's 292lbs (21 stone). That's because Hopkins was playing one short period in Hitch's life – the time he was filming *Psycho*.

In fact, he had enjoyed a slim period after moving to Hollywood in the 1940s – despite taking his personal cook with him. There's an interesting article[15] on the website of the Harry Ransom Center at the University of Texas at Austin that sheds some light on Hitch's massive weight-loss – said to be around 100lbs.

---

[15] http://blog.hrc.utexas.edu/2013/12/02/fellows-find-hitchcocks-weight

The author of the article researched Hitch's experiences as an obese man and how they influenced his film-making. He initially thought that the body standards of Hollywood had been imposed on Hitch by people such as the producer David O Selznick. Once he started researching, though, he discovered the opposite - that Selznick had actually used Hitch's obesity as a marketing ploy. Selznick realized that Hitch stood out, he was more memorable precisely because of his size. In one publicity shot organized by Selznick, Hitch is pictured holding a massive fake barbell, another is captioned '239 Englishman'.

When Selznick heard about Hitch's weightloss, he sent him a note:

> **'Drink a malted!'**

Using Hitch's obesity for publicity didn't stop Selznick also doing what we would call 'fat shaming' though. He would make snide comments about Hitch's big appetite, ask how his metabolism was, and say he was getting 'too big for his britches'. Nasty.

Most writers who have researched Hitch's life and works agree that he had a complicated relationship with food. He told an interviewer once:

> *'I'm frightened of eggs. That white round thing without any holes... have you ever seen anything more revolting than an egg yolk breaking and spilling its yellow liquid?'*

Hitch didn't just eat, he gorged – turning mealtimes into mini horror films that made anyone watching feel queasy. After a binge (and they were regular) he would be filled with self-loathing and embark on crash diets.

It was on one of his crash diets that he lost the massive amount of weight I mentioned earlier. He did that by eating melon, lean meat, and black coffee. That was an unsustainable way to eat - after the diet his weight ballooned again.

One of Hitch's biggest problems was the speed he ate. Those who saw him eat reported that he ate very quickly and didn't appear to chew much. This is very significant. We know now that eating quickly is disastrous for digestion and we aren't what we eat, we are what we digest and absorb.

The website Bon Appetit[16] records an interesting comment by comedian Mel Brooks. Brooks had dined with Hitch at Hitch's favorite restaurant.

---

[16] http://www.bonappetit.com/people/celebrities/article/mel-brooks-on-omelettes-coffee-and-the-inimitable-appetite-of-alfred-hitchcock

Brooks described the event:

> *'He had his own booth; he had his own waiter... he ordered a shrimp cocktail to begin, with cocktail sauce. And a sirloin steak, which was at least 2' thick. And a baked potato crammed full of chives and sour cream. And then he ordered a separate plate of asparagus with hollandaise sauce. And some sliced tomato on lettuce and there was some kind of blue cheese dressing on that... for dessert he had two bowls of vanilla ice cream with chocolate sauce, with strawberry or something on top.*
>
> *What a meal.'*

If that sounds shocking, what happened next is far more so.

After the meal, Hitch called over the head waiter:

> *The headwaiter ran over and Hitch said, 'George, I'm really peckish tonight. Do it again.'*

Now that's really shocking!

Hitch's complicated relationship with food may have had multiple causes – physical and psychological. Cravings and binging can be caused by deficiencies, as the body cries out for nutrients.

They can also be due to various psychological things:

> Childhood memories – we often crave foods that gave us comfort as children: ice cream, cake, soda.

> Stress – certain foods, carbohydrates in particular, act on the brain in the same way that heroin does. When we eat them, we get a similar feel-good feeling. We tend to seek out high-energy foods to get this endorphin high. Hitch had a lifelong love of ice cream and it was one of his cravings – usually late at night. It may have evoked memories and feelings of childhood: security, freedom from adult concerns, relaxation.

We know that Hitch had deep psychological problems – his films are testament to that – maybe his eating was an attempt to self-medicate and attain inner peace.

Author John Fawell comments that:

> *'In Hitchcock's films, eating often stands for the rottenness of humanity: the way humans consume things, break them down, dirty them, make them worse than they were. He saw a similar act of corruption in dinners, murders, and love relationships.'*

He also points out that food was rarely filmed in an appetizing way in Hitch's films. (Fawell, 2004)

Oh for a world-class psychiatrist!

Hitch's mental state was played out in his films, which became more tense as he grew more pessimistic. He feared what he felt was increasing evil in the world.

Some of the actors who worked with him dared to speculate that the great man himself had a touch of evil about him. Tippi Hedren, who famously acted in *The Birds*, claimed that he ruined her career after she rejected him sexually[17]. She said:

> *'I think he was an extremely sad character. We are dealing with a brain here that was an unusual genius, and evil, and deviant, almost to the point of dangerous, because of the effect that he could have on people that were totally unsuspecting.'*

One of his other leading ladies referred to his 'sadistic sense of humor' and a playwright recalled that Hitch was always...

> *'Engrossed in thinking up wicked practical jokes to play on the more vulnerable artists'.*
>
> Spoto, 2009

He's an interesting character because of this streak of darkness. He liked to embarrass his actresses and used

[17] http://www.dailymail.co.uk/news/article-2182804/Hitchcock-star-Tippi-Hedren-says-director-evil-shed-rich-sexual-harassment-laws-applied-1960s.html

bawdy language that shocked them.

His personal life, though, was mostly calm and ordered. (One exception was a dreadful time when he left his daughter alone, trapped and screaming at the top of a ferris wheel.) He wore a uniform of dark suits and white shirts and loved reading. He had a quirky habit of telling stories in elevators and leaving just before the punchline, loving the intrigued looks of the people he was leaving behind!

Hitch was bossy with his actors but it seems to have been the other way around at home. In *Spellbound by Beauty* (Spoto, 2009), Alma comes across as 'peppery and given to bossing her husband', a statement the author says was confirmed by one of Hitch's granddaughters.

The book points out that Alma seemed uneasy about Hitch's habit of playing pranks on people. She said:

> *'He never stopped playing jokes on people and now and then I got a little apprenehsive.'*

Their marriage appears to have been fairly celibate.

Hitch's Later Life & Death

After making around a film a year for most of his directing career, Hitch only made 6 films in the last 20 years of his life. He seemed to go downhill after being rejected by Tippi Hedren.

He had a history of drinking quite heavily and that worsened at this time. He was actually hospitalized for alcoholism at one point. He complained of loneliness but actually caused much of it himself, by firing longstanding workers. (Peele, 1986)

Hitch suffered from excruciating arthritis in later years and had cortisone injections to help the pain. He also had a heart condition, as he had a pacemaker.

Considering his lifelong battle with his weight and psychological problems, he lived to a surprisingly good age – 80. He had been declining for a year, suffering kidney failure.

He was interviewed[18] by the UK's BBC for a popular radio show, *Desert Island Discs*. On this show, the guest lists the books, music, and luxury item they would choose to have with them if they had to live on a desert island for any length of time. It's very significant that the book Hitch chose was *Mrs Beeton's Book of Household Management* – a cookbook.

What Can We Learn From Hitch?

GET HELP

For all his filmmaking genius, Hitch had some serious psychological problems. The evil that people who

---

[18] The interview took place before *Psycho* was released. Hitch referred to it as a 'rather gentle horror' that he was planning.
http://the.hitchcock.zone/wiki/Desert_Island_Discs_%28BBC_Radio,_19/Oct/1959%29_-_Alfred_Hitchcock

worked with him referred to may have been simple frustration from a sexless marriage, a form of revenge for childhood experiences, or something more serious.

Most of Hitch's biographers refer to his slightly weird relationship with his mother. After his father's death, his mother demanded a very close relationship with her son. We can perhaps read too much into his films but there has been a lot of speculation about the 'clinging, demanding' mother in *Psycho* (Bauso, 1994). Was this a portrayal or an exaggeration of his mother? We'll probably never know but it makes you wonder.

As an article on the *Neurophilosophy* website concludes:

> *'Freud would have concluded that Hitchcock's attitude towards women, and his obsession with strong mother figures, is probably due to Hitchcock's experiences of his own mother, who sometimes made the young Hitchcock stand at the foot of her bed for several hours as a punishment (this is alluded to in a scene in Psycho).'*

Whatever it was, it doesn't look like he sought help for it. Instead, he projected his own problems onto the roles his actors played. Men often played accomplished men who were overly attached to their mothers and uncertain of their own abilities. Women were the objects of his frustration, desire, and anger.

Most writers believe Hitch was haunted by a sense of

his own unattractiveness and that Tippi Hedren's rejection of him had a devastating effect.

Hitchcock's treatment of Tippi, however, was far worse.

EAT SLOWLY

Fellow diners commented that Hitch ate very quickly. He barely had time to chew. Eating quickly is known to be bad for digestion (chewing releases digestive enzymes which help to break down food before it even reaches the stomach). There's another important reason not to scarf down our food speedily. When we see and smell our food, digestion begins.

> *'First, even before you take a bite, your eyes, your sense of smell, and even your imagination are preparing you for the treat to come: The salivary glands in your mouth begin to produce saliva in anticipation. (If you doubt the power of your mind to affect your digestion, try just thinking about chewing on a piece of fresh lemon, and notice the extra saliva in your mouth!) As you put food into your mouth, the saliva is ready to work, moistening the food to make it easier for the teeth to grind into smaller pieces for swallowing.'*
>
> Norton Greenberger

DON'T CRASH DIET

Hitch spent his life either binging or crash dieting. One

of the effects of unbalance like that is a ruined metabolism, which makes gaining even more weight much easier and losing it far harder.

If you find yourself craving certain things and/or binging there are a couple of things you can do:

- ➢ Run your diet through a nutrient checker such as MyFitnessPal. If you are deficient in one or more nutrients, your cravings could be related to that. So if you are deficient in magnesium, for example, you could crave chocolate because that contains magnesium. Try eating more green vegetables, seeds, beans, lentils, and avocadoes and you should find your craving for chocolate lessens and eventually disappears.

- ➢ Consider potassium. It is one of the nutrients that many of us are deficient in and it has huge benefits. Eat things like bananas, beans, green veg, avocados.

- ➢ See a specialist for counseling. Binging and craving can be signs of psychological problems. People sometimes develop addictions (i.e. to food) as a way to help them through something. The trouble is that, while an addiction can help a person through a short-term problem, it can be destructive long-term. So, while an addiction may help you feel better for a while, it could ultimately kill you. Only a specialist in addictions or eating disorders could have the skills to help you through that. The 'Psychology of Eating' website can be helpful in the meantime. They have an excellent article[19] on different types of cravings and the psychological drives that can be behind them.

➢ A book that could help is *Brain over Binge* by former bulimic Kathryn Hansel. She has an unusual approach that works for many people.

---

[19] http://psychologyofeating.com/3-types-of-cravings/

'Mama' Cass Elliot

Crash dieting can kill

Cass Elliot, or 'Mama Cass', was born Ellen Naomi Cohen in 1941. She trained on piano and guitar but it was only later on that she realized what a good voice she had, becoming one of the huge stars of her generation in the group 'The Mamas & The Papas'.

She had a big personality, superstar charisma, and brilliant sense of humor that fooled people into thinking she was comfortable with herself and her weight. In fact she wasn't - she spent much of her life trying to lose weight, often through prolonged fasting. She mocked herself and took the jokes made about her in good spirit but she was simply absorbing the pain and not dealing with it and letting it out.

When she died, aged just 32, the rumormill kicked in straightaway and word spread that she had choked to death on a sandwich. She hadn't, her heart gave out due to years of obesity and crash dieting.

Cass's Early Life & Health

Cass was born in Baltimore to Bess and Philip Cohen. They were accomplished and musical people. Bess was a nurse who had been a professional singer and Philip a businessman and opera lover.

Their heritage was Jewish Russian. Both sets of Cass's grandparents were part of a large number of Jews who left Russia in the late 19th century.

Cass claimed that she was able to speak five languages by the age of four – but that would be an exaggeration. What was true was her incredible IQ – 165. She learned to speak at the age of just 6 months and to read by the time she was 2.

She was an only child until she was eight, when her sister was born, followed by a brother three years later. As a result of those years as an only child, she was able – like many only children – to converse with adults at a mature level and enjoyed political debate. This, and her desire to overcome people's objections to her weight, caused her to have a lively and forceful personality.

We don't know very much about her eating habits as a child but we do know that she was overweight by the age of seven so there was an early problem. She later admitted that being fat (her word) set her apart from others. But she also said:

> **'I'm going to be the most famous
> fat girl who ever lived.'**

This was in the 50s and 60s, when America didn't yet have a national weight problem - obesity was not as common as it is now and Cass was an intriguing oddity. According to her biographer Eddi Fiegel, Cass's size 'made her the object of derision and abuse.' (Fiegel, 2006)

Cass learned a lot from her mother and grandmother, who were also strong women. They were unusual for their era – both going out to work at a time when it was customary for women to remain at home.

While she was in high school she changed her name to Cass and later on changed her surname to Elliot in memory of a deceased friend.

Her family had financial difficulties throughout her childhood, including multiple bankruptcies. They moved around a lot, due to her father's work in mobile restaurant businesses.

Music was a big part of family life. Cass said[20] that the whole family would gather around the piano and sing together. Her sister later went on to also become a professional singer.

Cass got the acting bug in high school, after being in a production of *The Boy Friend*, and moved to NYC after leaving school. She did different jobs between acting work – including one that would prove useful, as a cloakroom attendant at a club. The club would sometimes allow her to sing.

---

[20] Interview on the Mike Douglas Show

She still pursued her acting ambitions and landed several off-Broadway roles. One of her 'failures' was on a part in a musical that went to Barbra Steisand! It was her singing that was to give her incredible success though. In the words of one tribute, she:

> ***Burst onto the early '60s
> Greenwich Village folk scene.***

She had success in a number of groups and married one of her bandmates in 1963. It may not have been a love-match – rumor said it was merely to help him avoid being drafted into the Vietnam war and the marriage was never consummated.

She later followed a former bandmate and joined a group called the New Journeymen but it took her a while to convince them to let her join. The story for years was that one of the group members, John Elliot, felt her vocal range was too small[21] but the truth eventually emerged – he thought she was too fat.

Eventually, John realized that her phenomenal voice was what they needed in the band, which had by then changed its name to The Mamas & The Papas. Cass joined them in 1965 and they had a series of big hits. Being called Cass, it was a natural thing for people to refer to her as Mama Cass – but she disliked it. She tried but was unable to stop her fans from using the

---

[21] Mama Cass confirmed a rumor that her vocal range increased after a concussion but this may have been to cover up the fact that John felt she was too fat to join the band

name, even after releasing an album called 'Don't Call Me Mama Cass Anymore'.

Life in the band wasn't easy. It was made up of husband and wife John & Michelle Phillips, Denny Doherty, and Cass. Michelle and Denny had an affair, which John found out about. Cass fell in love with Denny. It must have been complicated and, no doubt, stressful!

Les Macdonald, writing about the tension in the band in his book *The Day The Music Died* said the band was:

> *[The band] was beginning to crack from the internal pressure of the various relationships in the band.'*

Whatever the internal pressures were like, people still liked Cass. A good friend who knew her well said:

> *'I will give you a hundred dollars if you can find a single person who says they hated Cass.'*
>
> David Crosby to author Eddi Fiegel.

Fiegel, after interviewing over a hundred people who knew Cass, didn't earn his $100.

Cass went on to be even more successful after leaving The Mamas & The Papas. She appeared in films, TV, and sang at sold-out performances. She even showed off her comedy skills by hosting The Tonight Show several times.

What Went Wrong For Cass?

REJECTION

Sadly, we don't know very much about her childhood eating habits (other than that **may** have been fond of cookies[22]) or what really caused her early weight problems. What we do know is that the family moved around a lot and that she said being fat set her apart from others.

We don't know if the stress of moving and having to settle into different schools numerous times caused her to comfort eat.

From the research I have done into the people who made the pages of this book, I've noticed that weight problems generally have several causes – both physical and psychological.

Let's look at the facts for Cass:

- ➢ She was highly intelligent
- ➢ She was able to talk easily with adults as a child
- ➢ She had musical talent and an impressive voice
- ➢ She was regularly the 'new girl' at school
- ➢ She was Jewish

I can't imagine the High School mean girls and boys welcoming her with open arms. I can imagine them whispering about her, trying to put her down in order to make themselves seem more popular/intelligent,

---

[22] When asked if she had a childhood nickname, Cass said it was 'Cookie' (the Mike Douglas show interview)

and that causing deep psychological scars for Cass and they could even have caused her to start binging and fasting.

She experienced rejection in adulthood as well – due to her weight. She once told fellow Mama Michelle Phillips:

> *'Fat girls need love too'*

Denny Doherty described her first meeting with John Philips, the other 'Papa' in the band. He said:

> *'Cass arrived wearing a pink angora sweater, a little white pleated skirt and matching go-go boots. John looks at her, 'Jesus, what is that?''*

Ow. Cass didn't appear (on the surface) to be offended at the comment. She entered the room, introduced herself and gave everyone what she called 'pressies' (presents) – LSD-laced sugar cubes. They ate them.

DRUGS

My mother was in the entertainment industry during this period, she was a singer with the big bands. She left because of the drug problem, it was everywhere.

Many well-known people died way too early because of the drug culture in those years, others ruined their health and looks.

We know that Cass indulged – it would have been bigger news if she hadn't. It is likely that the drugs further damaged her metabolism, as well as her brain, leading to uncontrolled cravings and energy problems.

BINGING & FASTING

Cass was known for having a great sense of humor so it's unfair to take everything she said as gospel truth and she certainly wasn't afraid to mock herself or tease journalists. She did, however, make an interesting comment to one journalist that could be a hint at a struggle with bulimia:

> *'I'm ravenous. I threw up everything I ate last night.'* [23]

That could well have been a sarcastic reaction to hurtful press speculation but there's often a grain of truth in throw-away comments.

The other big thing that may have been an issue was alcohol. Bandmate Denny Doherty's website has several mentions in its stories from those days of drinking sessions he and Cass had together. The two of them would 'crack open a bottle of Jack Daniels'[24] and even on their first meeting there was drink involved as

---

[23]   http://www.newspapers.com/newspage/17984687/
[24]   http://www.dennydoherty.com/dream/dream18.html

Cass said:

> *'We're going to try and drink each other under the table aren't we? So let's get under the table and drink.'*

In 1968, after leaving The Mamas & The Papas, Mama Cass got a great gig – three weeks headlining at Caesars Palace in Las Vegas. It was a big deal and she was determined to look good and be strong and healthy enough to get through the rehearsals and two shows a night. So she went on a six-month diet – a crash diet. The result was a massive 100lb weight loss but also a stomach ulcer and throat problems severe enough to affect her wonderful voice.

She lost another large amount of weight just before her death. Fasting four days a week over a period of eight months produced an 80lb weight loss. It could also have affected her heart, as it was a heart attack[25] that killed her – at the age of just 32.

Anorexics and bulimics - and others who fast or severely restrict their food intake - often suffer from heart problems. It's caused by not eating enough. When we don't eat enough to fuel normal bodily needs, the body will take the fuel from the body itself, including muscles, which are a rich source of nutrients. As the heart is a muscle, that's one of the things that will be used up – with fatal consequences.

---

[25] The official cause was 'fatty myocardial degeneration due to obesity '.

One of the most famous people killed by anorexia was another singer and another person who died at the age of 32 - Karen Carpenter. Karen had also yo-yo dieted and had periods of both losing and gaining weight quickly. It all puts strain on the heart, even though Karen was never anything like as big as Cass.

According to the National Eating Disorders website[26], the binge/purge cycles that bulimics go through affect the entire digestive system, leading to electrolyte and chemical imbalances in the body. These imbalances can affect the heart, as well as other major organs, leading to irregular heartbeats and eventual heart failure.#

Even if Cass wasn't bulimic, she did have binging and fasting tendencies, which are remarkably similar. They probably weakened her heart, as well as other organs.

Her weight fluctuated a lot over the years as she tried diet after diet to try to control it. Many of them were experimental and dangerous – including trying drugs.

In the last couple of years of her life she seemed much more content to those around her.

What We Can Learn From Cass

EAT REGULAR MEALS

Like many performers, Cass lived on the road a lot, performing late at night and eating afterwards. What's open at midnight? Not much, just fast food places.

---

[26] http://www.nationaleatingdisorders.org

If you are able to keep regular mealtimes it is much better for your health than just grabbing food whenever the mood takes you. Because that's just it – you'll start to eat because of mood, not because of hunger or regularity of routine. Moods are erratic and unreliable and not a reliable method of deciding what and when to eat.

If your body starts to realize that you are going to feed it every morning shortly after you wake, at lunchtime, and in the evening, it won't have to ask you continually by giving you cravings and hunger pangs.

Having regular mealtimes can also lead to other regularity – particularly of the bathroom kind! That in itself can be a health boost. Becoming constipated can kick off other problems – pain, bad breath, flatulence, depression – that can increase the likelihood of comfort eating. You don't have to put up with such a vicious circle. You can turn it on its head to become a spiral of increasing health.

FIND WAYS TO DEAL WITH STRESS

Stress is a big cause of weight problems – both weight gain and inability to lose fat.

Many medical and obesity experts are fond of pointing out that stress raises levels of the hormone cortisol in the body. Cortisol is actually a steroid hormone (a little like adrenaline) which is released when we are under stress, to help us cope. Unfortunately, it also helps us gain weight. Studies[27] have been done using cortisol injections and the study participants experienced increased hunger, sugar cravings, and weight gain. Researchers noticed that the cortisol injections caused people to eat more foods high in fat and sugar and said it was due to cortisol binding to certain receptors in the brain.

Supplements such as Cortislim™ promise to help people lose weight by stopping some of the fat-boosting effects of cortisol – but without helping people deal with the causes of the stress!

Tips for dealing with stress:

> **Exercise** – love it or loathe it, exercise does have important stress-reduction benefits. The good news is that you don't have to take up running, which is actually stressful on the body. Gentle exercise is far better. Think swimming, Pilates, walking, and anything that puts a smile on your face!

> **Eat well** – some foods actually put the body into stress. Sugar is a well-known one but really it is very individual. Many of us have foods that just don't agree with us. Find out what yours are by noticing what goes on in your mind and body during and after eating, keeping a food diary, or doing the pulse test[28].

---

[27] http://www.unm.edu/~lkravitz

[28] A pulse test is useful for determining which foods your body reacts to in some way but it isn't a medical test. Don't rely on it to tell you about a food *allergy*. Food allergies can be life-threatening and only

➤ **Get enough sleep** – our fast-paced, always-available culture treats the hours 'lost' to sleep as an irritating inconvenience. If we could start to see them as a huge health benefit, we would all feel a lot better.

The National Sleep Foundation points out in an 'Ask The Expert' article on their website[29] that stress causes insomnia by making it difficult to fall asleep and stay asleep. Many people only link waking in the early hours with depression, but stress is also a big cause.

So what can you do to reduce stress if stress is causing insomnia, which increases stress?! Sleep experts recommend 'sleep hygiene' which is a bit old news really – keep the bedroom dark, don't watch TV in bed, keep regular hours, try a warm bath, blah, blah. The bottom line is that we need to find routines that agree with us. It may be that a computer/tablet habit is causing you to stay awake, or that your partner's snoring is a problem. Whatever it is, try doing something different in your evening routine every single day for a week and see if it makes a difference. If it doesn't, try something else, then something else. Sleep is so important that it pays to spend time on discovering and eliminating the problem.

Stress isn't the only thing that sleep helps. The Harvard School of Public Health reported[30] on a

proper medical tests are reliable at uncovering them.

[29] http://sleepfoundation.org/ask-the-expert/stress-and-insomnia
[30] http://www.hsph.harvard.edu/obesity-prevention-source/

number of studies that link lack of sleep to obesity. One showed that children who slept less than 10 and a half hours sleep a night had a 45% higher risk of becoming obese by the age of 7.

Just remember that too much sleep is as bad as too little. It's more about sleeping in time with the natural rhythms of nature. If it is light outside in the mornings, you would feel better if you got up and got outside. Lying in bed until mid-morning isn't the route to good health. Getting up early isn't easy if you aren't used to it. That's why you need to get your circadian rhythms in sync by getting natural daylight. When it goes dark, your mind and body will understand that it's coming up to bedtime, and start winding down. When it's light, it will start making you more energetic. It can take a couple of weeks but it's well worth the effort.

➢ **Don't resort to prescription drugs** - I once read an article that I thought helpful at the time, when I was suffering from Chronic Fatigue Syndrome. It pointed out the importance of sleep in healing and said, 'Take whatever you have to in order to get 8 hours of sleep every night.'

The advice did help my fatigue, short-term (it returned with a vengeance) but it created a 5-year sleeping tablet dependency. That dependency was incredibly hard to break. So I would caution you not to use drugs, even prescription drugs (see the chapter on Elvis if you aren't convinced) in order to improve your sleep quality/duration. Instead try herbal teas, aromatherapy oils/massages, blackout curtains, computer software such as Flu.x[31] (which gradually reduces the intensity of the brightness of computer screens once it gets to dusk).

START BELIEVING THAT EATING IS GOOD

So many people, affected by our appearance-led culture, seem to feel that they are doing 'well' if they don't eat very much. In fact, they could be causing long-term problems for themselves.

If we don't eat enough calories, our bodies will find other ways to get them (including, as mentioned earlier, raiding muscles). The body will also reduce the need for calories so it doesn't have to go shopping in muscle fibers too often. People who don't eat enough feel energetic at first, because eating uses up a lot of energy. After a short period, though, they find themselves crashing, energy-wise, and struggling to get through the day. They also find that their hair starts to lose its luster and texture, their skin stops looking healthy, and they generally begin to get depressed. This is all because the body has diverted its small source of calories into things that are vital for life – and it doesn't think shining hair is too important!

Humans need around 1,500 calories a day just for vital cellular functions. So if you were lying in bed for a

---

[31] https://justgetflux.com

week, after an injury, you would need 1,500 calories a day for your body to do its repair work, as well as its regular tasks relating to breathing, sleeping, digestion, cellular repair and growth, lymphatic work, detoxing, and much else. Add exercise and work to your day and your need for calories goes up.

People who exist on 600 calories a day when crash dieting are doing untold damage, not only to their bodies in the here and now but to their future weight, because the body will quickly go into starvation mode and reduce the need for calories, leading to weight gain as soon as a more normal diet is resumed.

Getting to a place of acceptance that food is vital for health is hugely important. There's a massive difference between 1,500 calories of high quality foods such as fruits, vegetables, pulses, nuts, and seeds and 1,500 calories of donuts and cakes. While we do need calories, we need them to come loaded with nutrients, not loaded with sugar and fat.

DON'T EAT YOUR EMOTIONS

Cass experienced rejection in a lot of areas: from children at school; from potential bands; and from the press. All caused by her weight.

It's no wonder that she developed her well-known 'big' personality and covered up her feelings. But, actually, that really wasn't helpful. Covering up our feelings causes us to deal with them in other ways – sometimes by comfort eating, sometimes by even more harmful things such as self-harm through cutting and risky behaviors.

Finding other ways to deal with emotions is far healthier, especially long-term. Counseling, assertiveness classes, exercise, and simple honesty can all help.

A lady I knew who had suffered terribly from Chronic Fatigue Syndrome said that the turning point for her was learning assertiveness. She is finally – in middle age – able to stand up for herself, in gentle and polite ways, and not do things that go against her sensitivities (e.g. watching horror films with her husband), eat things that don't agree with her (e.g. refusing food at dinner parties by letting the hosts know well in advance), or take on board other people's rubbish and problems (setting time limits on telephone calls from moaning friends and lightly distancing herself from people who continually bring her down). That means she isn't internalizing hurt and frustration, and deals with emotions as they come up. It's a far healthier situation.

It's sad that many people get to old age before they learn to stop worrying about what other people think. They make great oldies but they waste a lot of years!

ACCEPT YOURSELF

Learning to accept yourself with all your quirks can be the most amazing thing you can do. It can revolutionize your life in ways you can't begin to imagine.

Cass must have really struggled with the reaction of

everyone, throughout her life, to her weight. A friend said after her death:

> *'I don't think Cass was ever happy... inside she was very beautiful but our society is built on surface not substance... she never talked about it or came out front but she wanted to be beautiful! She wanted to be loved. I think that was probably the single greatest driving force in her character.'*
>
> David Crosby. (Fiegel, 2006)

In the interview on the Mike Douglas Show, Cass was asked if she was a precocious child. She replied:

> *'Yes. Nasty too.'*

She had a strong, loving family, intelligence, world-class talent, and a massive number of adoring fans yet she referred to herself in negative ways.

Over-honesty and complete transparency can be a sign of an insecure person. It's the 'shoot first' mentality – we think if we point out our own faults we leave less for others to notice.

I hope Cass was only declaring her supposed nastiness to get a laugh on the show. It's sad to think that she may have believed herself to be an unlovable person when the opposite was actually the case. It is probably the case for most of us.

Marlon Brando

Don't eat your emotions – deal with them

What does the name 'Brando' conjure up for you? Most people think of an angry, hard-drinking working class man – the stereotypical role he often played. But he was so much more than that, as well as a true Method actor who *became* his characters.

He enjoyed early success after learning his craft on the New York circuit. He studied in classes and workshops, and took small parts in stage productions. His talent and presence drew attention early on. He became popular with theatre-goers and was spotted by talent scouts. He was determined to learn his craft thoroughly and even turned down several film roles. That was probably also due to not wanting to be tied to one studio for their standard seven-year contracts.

His first major role was also one of his biggest – Stanley Kowalski in *A Streetcar Named Desire*. He won Best Actor in the Academy Awards for that role and went on to win seven more. He inspired many other actors, including Elvis Presley and James Dean. In fact, the website Internet Movie Database notes that:

> *No actor ever exerted such a profound influence on succeeding generations of actors as did Brando.*

His stellar career was almost – but not quite – eclipsed by his car-wreck of a private life. Numerous marriages, problems with his children, and endless battles with his weight scarred his life. The reasons for these all stem from his childhood, as we will see.

Brando's Early Life

Marlon Brando (his real name, he was 'Bud' to his family though) was one of three children born into an unhappy home in Omaha in 1924[32]. His mother was an melancholic, frustrated actress. She blamed her husband for her failed acting career but her excessive drinking could have had more to do with it.

She was very involved in amateur dramatics and became a director of the Omaha Community Playhouse. One website[33] insists that during that time she mentored Henry Fonda. When she wasn't busy with her dramatic ambitions she was frequently drunk. This

---

[32] http://www.manythings.org/voa/people/Marlon_Brando.html

[33] http://www.lifetimetv.co.uk/biography/biography-marlon-brando

wasn't just the occasional social drinking session - she was often picked up by the local police.

Perhaps due to her regular incompetence, the family employed at least one nanny. Brando had a troubling relationship with one when he was very young – they shared a bed, naked. Many biographers feel this odd relationship prompted his lifelong fascination with ethnic women – the nanny was Danish-Indonesian.

Brando gave an interesting insight into his early relationship with food in his autobiography, *Brando: Songs My Mother Taught Me*:

> *'When I was a kid, I'd come home from school to find my mother gone and the dishes in the sink. I'd feel low and open the icebox, and there would be an apple pie, along with some cheese, and the pie would say: 'C'mon, Marlon, take me out. I'm freezing in here. Be a pal and take me out, and bring out Charlie Cheese, too.' Then I'd feel less lonely.'*

Young Brando's father (also called Marlon) was a traveling salesman who also had a drinking problem. The effects of his father's drinking on Brando were worse than those caused by his mother, as his father was an angry drunk who took his frustrations out on his son.

His parents separated for a while but got back together, although their arguments continued. It had an effect on young Brando, he constantly got into trouble at school. A classmate recalled that he 'drummed on everything', indicating a nervous tic early on. He was eventually expelled for riding a motorbike through the school halls.

Eventually, Brando's father sent him to military school, which did little to help him either academically or behaviorally (he was expelled). It did spark his interest in acting though and he headed to New York to further his interest. He was actually following in the footsteps of his sister Jocelyn, who had also headed to New York to pursue an acting career. He opted for acting because it was the only thing he had ever received praise for.

He took acting classes and discovered a love for Method acting. He had a natural flair for it and landed parts in numerous plays. His first major role was in a Broadway play several years after moving to New York. The play was *A Streetcar Named Desire'* – quite a breakthrough role at the age of just 23.

He later starred in the movie version of Desire – and played similar roles at times for the rest of his career as hard drinking, brutal, working-class men.

Brando's Early Health

We don't know much about Brandon's childhood health. We can assume it wasn't bad – otherwise there would be mentions in his numerous biographies.

In his early film roles, he looks amazing. His skin glows and his muscles ripple. That incredible physique didn't last for long, though. People who worked with him even in his early years were commented on his poor eating habits then.

Richard Erdman, one of his colleagues on his first film commented that Brando's daily diet was:

> *Junk food, take out, and peanut butter.*[34]

When Erdman said peanut butter, he meant whole jars of the stuff – jars and jars. Brando was also known for eating whole boxes of cereal and drinking quarts of milk.

He would also eat boxes of biscuits and cakes, not one or two things, and accompany them with an entire quart of milk.

His weight bothered him and he started a lifelong dieting rollercoaster - going on extreme diets, then giving up and binging. His snacks became legendary: a pound of bacon in a whole loaf of bread; stacks of pancakes swimming in maple syrup; 5-gallon tubs of ice cream; six hot dogs.

The effects of his appalling diet soon started to show. His appearance changed dramatically. It didn't make it easy for the people he worked for - costumes frequently had to be altered during filming. During the filming of *Mutiny on the Bounty* in 1962 (when he was

---

[34] http://www.todayifoundout.com/index.php/2012/11/
the-odd-eating-habits-of-marlon-brando

38), he allegedly split 52 pairs of trousers due to his weight fluctuations. Directors took to employing body doubles for him, in case he went on his lunchtime gorges.

Brando's Later Health

Despite critical acclaim and some hailing Brando as the greatest actor who ever lived, he was obviously deeply troubled. He built up a reputation for being difficult to work with. He nearly didn't get his most famous role in *The Godfather*, because of that. But Director, Francis Ford Coppola, insisted on Brando – and it resulted in him winning the Best Actor Oscar.

Brando's professional life was phenomenally successful (especially in the early years) but his personal life was the polar opposite. Brando's biographer Stefan Kanfer wrote:

> *'He abandoned all three wives and numerous lovers, often in fear that they would abandon him first. He loved his eleven children but never knew how to relate to them once they entered adolescence – a shortcoming that would have fatal consequences.'*

Kanfer speculated that Brando's later weight problems were the result of his discomfort with fame and the attention he received when his celebrity grew. Men and women found him attractive and pursued him relentlessly. Kanfer believed that Brando felt:

> *'The more beguiling his appearance,*
> *the less comfortable he was with it,*
> *finally distancing himself from his*
> *admirers by putting on weight until*
> *he grew morbidly obese.'*

His weight fluctuated due to binges and crash dieting. At one point he weighed over 300lbs. Even after becoming diabetic, he still continued his regular binges. Stories abound of his legendary binges, from friends and colleagues.

One of his wives resorted to locking the refrigerator door after their maid told her Brando would raid the refrigerator every night. The lock didn't stop him – she found it broken next morning and teeth marks in the cheese.

Brando would also drive out to hot dog places in the early hours of the morning, eating half a dozen at once.[35] He would eat so much during film shoots that directors got used to having to pull in body doubles – especially after lunch – and have the costume department on hand.

Directors were frequently shocked at his size when he appeared for the first time on set. This led to lots of close-up and dark shots of him, trying to disguise his weight.

---

[35] http://www.chimesdesign.com/blog/2012/04/15/on-binging-and-brando

He would frequently promise directors before shooting that he would lose weight, which he often did, only to regain it during shooting.

His wasn't a foodie, he would eat anything that took his fancy. Some stories claim that he had sacks of McDonald's cheeseburgers delivered to his Hollywood home.

His main culinary downfall was ice cream. Ice cream is a good example of one of the food combinations that can become addictive. It contains large amounts of both fat and sugar. Together these act like a drug on the brain.

An interesting documentary by the BBC aired in the UK around the time I was researching this book. They had a pair of twins eating either a low fat (high carb style) or a low sugar (Atkins style) diet and looked at the results. The result was not that either sugar or fat were the main problem when trying to lose weight, but rather that it is a combination of sugar and fat that is the big key.

Brando related many of his problems – not just his weight but also his womanizing – to his parents' drinking problems and his own stress eating.

Near the end of his life, he managed to lose 70lbs on another crash diet. That could have been the one that put the final strain on his heart.

Brando didn't come across, in his films, as a man of learning with a love of literature. So it was a surprise to many that he had a library of over 4,000 well-read books. Part of the reason for his huge library was the fact that he thoroughly researched every role he played, throughout his life.

His library also contained lots of self-help and psychology books. Many were on dieting. He once admitted:

> *'There probably isn't a diet I haven't tried.'*

What Went Wrong For Brando?

Brando's parents' alcohol problems had a severe effect on him. His mother's was due to her frustrated ambitions, his father just seems to have been a brute. Brando later wrote that his father never had anything good to say about him. He was scarred by his father's repeated assertions that his son would never amount to anything. A lifetime of success and critical acclaim would later fail to heal those wounds and he remained angry at his father until his own death.

Life at home must have been difficult for Brando: his parents' drinking; his mother's frustration; his father's consorting with prostitutes on his frequent travels; his father's violence towards him.

Brando used the emotions in his acting, saying:

> *'If I have a scene to play and I have
> to be angry, I can remember
> my father hitting me.'*

One of his biographers[36] wrote that:

> *'Brando's early years disfigured the rest
> of his life. He never fully emerged from
> the shadows of a cold and brutal father
> and a longing, desperately unhappy
> mother who squandered the best hours
> of her best years in an alcoholic haze.'*

Psychologists aren't surprised when children from dysfunctional homes act up. They are stressed from both the atmosphere at home and their need to keep up an appearance of everything being normal outside the home. In the book *Somebody*, author Stefan Kanfer quotes Gary Lefer, MD, a psychiatrist:

> *'Children of such parents live two lives:
> the false, well-kept one presented to
> the world at large, and the real and
> messy one that they know at home.
> They think they've put one over on their
> classmates, and thus know themselves to
> be phony. They grow up thinking that
> everything is bogus. Especially their own
> achievements.'*

---

[36] *Somebody*, Stefan Kanfer

One Brando's most recent biographers is Susan Mizruchi, who wrote *Brando's Smile: His Life, Thought And Work*.

She explains that, after going through the effects of his parents' volatile marriage and separation, he wanted to be a good father himself. He never felt that he achieved that though.

Muzruchi paints a sad portrait of him at the end of his life:

> *'Brando was guilt-ridden by his own failings. He feared that his own indulgent lifestyle had made life difficult for his children. He was a compassionate and caring father but never gave his children a stable family or the time they needed ... He was destroyed by his son's arrest and daughter's suicide. Towards the end of his life he was very depressed and felt he'd failed Cheyenne and Christian.'*

What a sad ending for the man who set the standard for acting. The man who Marilyn Monroe called *'The sexiest man in the world'.*

His sexuality was part of the problem though. He was a terrible womanizer, never truly finding peace and love in a relationship. He was on a path of self-destruction in so many ways, caused by hurts from his past. As fellow actor Anthony Quinn once said to Brando's first wife:

> *'I admire Marlon's talent,*
> *but I don't envy the pain that created it.'*

One of the things that surprised me when I researched Brando's life was his close relationship with Michael Jackson. Brando's son Miko (a close friend of Jackson) told an interview that Jackson's Neverland ranch was his father's 'second home'.

Brando found happiness at Neverland – not least because of the 24-hour availability of food! – and Miko said of his father's relationship with the megastar:

> *'Michael was instrumental helping my father through the last few years of his life … Dad had a hard time breathing in his final days, and he was on oxygen much of the time … Michael got Dad a golf cart with a portable oxygen tank so he could go around and enjoy Neverland. They'd just drive around – Michael Jackson, Marlon Brando, with an oxygen tank in a golf cart.'[37]*

Brando died at the age of 80 from lung failure. At the end he was also suffering from pulmonary fibrosis, congestive heart failure, and cancer.

---

[37] http://*larrykinglive*.blogs.cnn.com/2009/06/29/lkl-web-exclusive-michael-jacksons-friend-and-marlon-brandos-son-on-the-michael-jackson-he-knew

What Can We Learn From Brando?

THE 'ALL-OR-NOTHING' APPROACH DOESN'T WORK

Like many of the people featured in this book, Brando had an 'all-or-nothing' approach to periods of dieting and non-dieting. When he was dieting he would eat little, mostly bland foods. He would get so tired of that that he would crack and have a huge binge – often involving the five-gallon tubs of ice cream he so loved. Then, because he had broken his diet, he was off it so ate as much as he wanted. And he wanted to eat a lot. He had an addiction to foods – especially the fatal combination of sugar and fat.

If we recognize that this approach doesn't work, we can move towards overcoming it. Breaking your diet doesn't mean you have to go all the way and eat the whole contents of the refrigerator. Giving in on the journey home and having a whole chocolate bar doesn't mean you have to then carry on and order a takeout for 6 and eat it yourself. Giving in now and then is actually a good thing as it makes dieting feel less harsh. Binging instead of dieting is extremely hard on the body, though, and it's really important to get out of the feast or famine rollercoaster.

MOVING PAST CHILDHOOD HURTS IS IMPORTANT

Late in his career, Brando formed a production company and named it Pennebaker Productions – after his mother's maiden name. His early acting skills were honed by trying to get his mother's attention during her hazy drinking sessions and he took up the career she loved. He seems to have been fond of her but found her hard to reach and he may have spent his whole life trying to escape that hurt.

Like many people, Brando spent much of his life trying to get over his childhood hurts. He may have been better trying to make sure he didn't put his own children through the hurts that he went through. Instead (again like many of us!) he repeated history and put his own children through rages, unsettled lifestyle, and divorces.

People who are successful in overcoming the limitations of their childhood are those who realize they can't change or undo the past and decide to move on and do better, whatever it takes.

FAT & SUGAR IS A DANGEROUS COMBINATION

We know that crash diets usually end in binges and those binges frequently involved high far and high sugar foodstuffs. Think donuts, ice cream, cookies, cakes, pastries.

That's the fat & sugar combination at work. It acts like a drug on the brain, calming anxiety, and soothing hurt feelings. It acts like a drug in another way as well – it can be very addictive.

If you are craving something while dieting, just make

sure it doesn't have that fat/sugar combination and you won't kick off this addiction.

BELIEVE IN YOURSELF

Whatever we are good at, we tend to devalue. Many of us don't think very highly of ourselves. So we think that if we are good at something it must be very easy and that everyone can do it. That generally isn't the case.

Brando never felt that acting was important or that he had real talent. He believed acting was nothing special as everyone did it all the time in their everyday life. So he felt life was all play-acting. He became very serious and disillusioned.

It's such a pity he was unable to see and appreciate his own talents. If he had, he may have been more grateful for them, easier to work with, and more satisfied with his life and work.

§℞

We'll look at another immensely talented man next, another person who found success at an early age, but who also lost his looks early on through over-indulging...

Elvis Presley

Prescription drugs are still drugs

After a 22-year career as one of the most famous people on the planet, Elvis suffered a tragic, slow decline and death.

He had been a lithe, stunningly attractive young man, performing almost acrobatic stage moves and coping with all the demands of his career. By the time of his death he was a bloated caricature of his former self, dragging himself around and spending nearly all his spare time in his bedroom.

Elvis's Early Life & Health

Elvis Aaron Presley[38] was born on January 8th, 1935. He should have been a twin, but his brother Jessie was

---

[38] He like his surname to be pronounced the southern way, PRESSley, not PREZley. Vernon actually spelled his name Pressley until after Elvis became famous.

born stillborn. The family lived in a poor neighborhood of Tupelo, Mississippi. For the rest of his life, Elvis would blame poverty for his brother's death. His father Vernon later said of their poverty:

> *"At that time there was almost nobody poorer than my wife Gladys and me ... poor we were but trash we weren't. There were times we had nothing to eat but corn bread and water. But we always had compassion for people ... We never put anybody down. Neither did Elvis."*

Part of the reason for their poverty was that they married when very young, without resources. They had eloped to get married, lying about their ages. Gladys was known for such impetuousness – a trait she passed on to her son.

Vernon built the family home himself after learning that Gladys was expecting. The house was without electricity or plumbing but was similar to others in the area so didn't stand out. They were so poor that they sometimes had to eat squirrel.

Elvis (named after his father's middle name) grew to be very close to his parents. Vernon said they had a wonderful, balanced family relationship. Elvis grew up with his extended family of grandparents, aunts, uncles, and cousins nearby.

He was an average student at school – although he did impress a teacher by singing a country song. Many people have reported that he struggled to fit in and was quite a loner.

After Vernon was sent to prison for fraud (he wrote a fraudulent check), Elvis and his mother went to live with relatives. She had been unable to keep up with payments on their modest shotgun[39] home.

Elvis showed an interest his uncle's guitar so Gladys somehow managed to buy him a used one for his birthday. His uncle, together with another uncle and the family's pastor, gave him guitar lessons. He enjoyed them but refused to sing in public.

Elvis later said:

> *'I took the guitar, and I watched people,*
> *and I learned to play a little bit.*
> *But I would never sing in public.*
> *I was very shy about it.'*

After Vernon was released from prison, he struggled to find work so the family moved to Memphis. Job prospects were better there but living accommodation was not. They moved into a room in a housing project with a shared bathroom and no cooking facilities.

The move meant Elvis had to go to another new school and he didn't fit in, again being regarded as a loner by others. Eventually he started taking his guitar with him,

---

[39] A small, narrow home, similar to a railroad apartment, usually around 12ft wide. They were popular house styles from the end of the Civil War to the 1920s but became symbols of poverty.

playing at lunchtimes. It didn't help him gain friends as he favored what they thought of as trashy hillbilly music.

He did make one friend, though, whose older brother was a local radio DJ, Mississippi Slim. Slim gave Elvis extra guitar lessons and even managed to get him slots for radio performances. Incapacitating stage fright stopped Elvis managing the first slot but he did the second.

Elvis started at the local high school, accompanied – to his embarrassment – by his mother, who liked to walk him to school. He struggled to fit in and remained an outsider, despite being popular with girls. Most students viewed him as being a mama's boy. One biographer described him as being:

> *'Wary, watchful, shy almost to the point of reclusiveness.'*
>
> (Guralnick, 2014)

He soaked up the local music scene, though. He was influenced by church songs, as well as country music mixed with rhythm and blues. It was a heady mixture and influenced him for the rest of his life.

His early jobs (while still at school) weren't huge successes – probably because his heart wasn't in it. He was fired as a cinema usher for spending too much time watching the movies, then spent a short time as a delivery driver.

He started to stand out, due to both his appearance (sideburns and slicked back hair) and his talent. He formed a group with a few other kids and they played in the housing complex where the Presleys lived.

Eventually he plucked up the courage to play outside the complex and played at a local show. He said afterwards:

> *'I wasn't popular in school ... I failed music – only thing I ever failed. And then they entered me in this talent show ... it was amazing how popular I became after that.'*

He cut his first record as a present for his mother. He simply walked into a record label's studio and asked if he could pay for some studio time. His biographer Peter Guralnick maintains that Elvis used the record label's studio rather than a local general store's record making facilities because he hoped to be discovered. He wasn't discovered but the studio secretary made a note of his name.

Rejections followed as he was told he would never make it as a singer. His luck was to change, though. The original record label where he recorded were on the lookout for 'a white singer with the negro sound and the negro feel'. They still had his name so they invited Elvis in to try out and played the resulting song on the radio. It was the station's listening audience who launched Elvis's career, as they rang the station in droves, asking who the amazing new singer was and asking for the song to be played again.

Elvis's Career Success

Success came in highs and lows after that. Even while playing alongside giants like Roy Orbison, Elvis failed an audition to join a talent scout TV show. His music was just too different – there was no way of classifying it. But he broke through at the young age of 20, signing with RCA. His debut album with RCA featured country, pop, R&B, and a new sound which had guitar as the lead instrument instead of piano ... and which came to be known as rock & roll.

He took on a manager against his parents' initial wishes. The manager was Colonel Tom Parker. Vernon and Gladys met Parker and said he seemed like a smart man but they didn't sign the necessary contracts (Elvis was under age). They later agreed to Parker managing Elvis, after a country singer gave him a good character witness. His parents' initial feelings were probably right – Parker proved untrustworthy.

Heartbreak Hotel was Elvis's first pop hit and it defined his sound. Audiences hearing him reacted in extreme ways – younger people cheering and screaming and older people loathing him.

J. Edgar Hoover, then director of the FBI, received a letter warning that Elvis was a danger to US security because of the effect his performances had on his fans.

Many critics – generally older people – hated him. The New York Times wrote that he had no singing ability; Steve Allen thought him talentless and absurd; the New York Daily News said popular music had reached its lowest depths; Ed Sullivan decided Elvis was 'unfit for family viewing'; Time magazine reported that he performed as 'if he had swallowed a jackhammer'. A Florida judge even got in on the negativity, ordering Presley to tone down his act.

Elvis's father said the "brutal attacks" by some critics upset his son but that he learned to shrug them off over time. He said Elvis always said, "Truth will prevail."

Worryingly, one of the reasons for some of the negative reaction was a strong undercurrent of racism. Elvis had been influenced by black music and dance. He was nicknamed 'Elvis the Pelvis' because of his gyrating dance moves – a name he hated, calling it:

> *'One of the most childish expressions
> I ever heard, coming from an adult.'*

So Elvis was surrounded on one side by screaming, adoring fans and on the other by irate critics. It must have been an odd situation to be in and it soon propelled him to national celebrity. Everywhere he played there were riots as the fans lost control.

Once the big money started rolling in, Elvis bought a mansion for himself and his parents: Graceland.

He was drafted into the US Army in 1958. According to other soldiers, he was keen to be just another soldier, if a very generous one. His mother died soon after – with Elvis, given compassionate leave, at her side. He took it badly, they had remained very close.

His Army stint ended in 1960 and he returned to performing. He had confessed to being concerned that his career was over but the screaming fans were as devoted as ever.

After nearly a decade of devoting himself to film-making, his record sales started to slow. He got married to a beautiful teenager, Priscilla, at this time – devastating fans who had held out hopes of a relationship with him! He managed to stage a comeback and regained his earlier success. People noted that he seemed nervous, at times, though.

He faced numerous threats, the most famous being one where the FBI became involved. He performed onstage with guns tucked in his boot and waistband while the threats were at their worst.

Elvis was in danger frequently during his career, because of the hysteria of his fans. The crowd would sweep over him, rocking cars he traveled in and tearing at his clothes if they could get near enough. His father once said that the fans were "as out of control as a lynch mob".

Elvis's Later Years & Health

Poignantly, one of the 'Memphis Mafia' (Elvis's employees and friends) said that Elvis would not have deteriorated the way he did had his beloved mother not died so young.

Elvis didn't really get to have later years either, dying before he reached middle age. The start of his decline coincided with the breakdown of his marriage. He had been having an affair and Priscilla revealed that she had too, as they had become increasingly distant. It still hit Elvis hard. One of his contemporaries called the divorce:

> **'A blow from which he never recovered.'**
> Joe Moscheo

The split from Priscilla seemed to send Elvis a little crazy. At one of his performances, four men rushed the stage. Security helped but Elvis dealt with one of them himself (he was a fan of Karate). But he got so angry that a physician was sent for to sedate him. It didn't work.

Elvis blamed the man Priscilla was seeing. He became paranoid, believing that Priscilla's boyfriend was trying to kill him. He raged for days about it and those near to him were very concerned. After several days of madness he calmed down and let it go. But his song choices in his later years were mainly about regret and loss.

It's no coincidence that the year of the divorce – 1973 – was also the year that Elvis started to really put on weight. His weight had fluctuated over the years but now it was becoming more than a slight problem.

He was generally at his heaviest when touring. His tour schedules were packed and pressured and this was when he also started having a problem with drugs.

After the divorce Elvis had a girlfriend but he also entertained a lot of female fans. Marty Lacker, Elvis's accountant, told an interviewer that on Friday and Saturday nights, Elvis used to let all the girls in who hung around the gates of Graceland. Lacker went one night and counted the girls there – 152. For someone who liked his privacy, Elvis entertained a lot of visitors!

Keeping up with his demanding schedule and his hectic social life must have been difficult and drugs would have helped. His rock & roll lifestyle wasn't totally to blame though - he first took amphetamines to help him stay awake during his Army days, when he was on duty.

Knowing that they worked, Elvis knew he could take them to help him get through his demanding stage routines and traveling schedules. They were legal and readily available as appetite suppressants.

One of the bodyguards told an interviewer:

> *We stayed wired up all the time. we didn't go to bed 'til late and it was tiring so we'd take a little speed the next day to stay awake next day. Then a lot of times we couldn't go to sleep because we were high so we took a sleeping pill to go to sleep. We lived that way for a long time. Luckily we were young, we could do it.*
>
> Joe Esposito

Elvis overdosed on barbiturates twice (on one occasion

ending up in a three-day coma) and was hospitalized due to an opioid addiction.

Vernon Presley later admitted that:

> *"Elvis did take medication of several kinds, but it was all prescribed. For a while, he took diet pills, but he gave them up ... because he was afraid of them."*

His first prescription from his favorite physician, 'Dr Nick' (Dr George C Nichopoulos), was to treat insomnia. Elvis had episodes of insomnia (as well as sleepwalking and nightmares) since childhood and they got worse after the death of his mother.

His insomnia was made worse by his use of amphetamines. It took powerful drugs to knock Elvis out and they would leave him tired next day, requiring more amphetamines to get him going. It was a vicious circle and would only get worse.

Dr Nick told an interviewer:

> *'Elvis's problem was that he didn't see the wrong in it. He felt that by getting it from a doctor, he wasn't the common everyday junkie getting something off the street. He was a person who thought that, as far as medications and drugs went, there was something for everything.'*

Those close to Elvis were as blind to the problem as Elvis himself, kidding themselves the drugs were fine because they were prescribed. The problem was that Elvis went to numerous doctors to get his prescriptions – none of them knowing about the others.

Dr Nick tried to control Elvis's increasing use of drugs and took to traveling with him, in order to stop him from visiting other doctors, who would give him whatever he asked for.

Elvis had a strong anti-drug stance and didn't believe that his growing prescription drug dependency was a problem. His father backed this up, saying that Elvis would never take "hard, illegal drugs" because he had seen what they had done to people he'd known. It was unfortunate that he didn't know anyone who had been killed by prescription drugs.

It started to be a noticeable problem when band members reported that Elvis was slurring and uncoordinated at times. The public realized something was wrong when his weight began to balloon and his performances deteriorated.

Fans complained that his concerts were too short (barely an hour in some places) and that they couldn't understand him either talking or singing.

What Went Wrong For Elvis

When some of Elvis's bodyguards – his close friends for many years – started to challenge Elvis about his drug problem, Vernon Presley fired them. The bodyguards later wrote a book, *Elvis: What Happened?*, which detailed his decline. It listed his health problems in detail and all seemed to be either caused or worsened by his drug problems. They included glaucoma, high blood pressure, liver damage, and bowel problems[40].

Vernon Presley confirmed the health problems and threw some light on his son's lifestyle, telling an interviewer:

> *"When he wanted to lose weight, [Elvis] did it by cutting down on his food or by giving it up entirely. In fact, he'd fasted for the final 24 hours of his life. He did take sleeping pills, because he felt that he needed eight to ten hours of sleep to perform well. The doctors discovered that he had some liver damage, a colon problem, and high blood pressure."*

Yet again, we see the strains on the body of the desperate overweight person trying fasting and crash diets to lose weight.

Elvis's autopsy revealed that there were 14 different drugs in his system at the time of his death. A massive amount – in fact, more than the coroner had ever seen in one person.

The drugs were all prescribed. Like many stars, Elvis had a pet doctor. In his case it was Dr Nick. He wrote 10,000 prescriptions in 1977, the year of Elvis's death.

---

[40] Constipation was a big problem but even Elvis's doctor didn't realize how big of a problem until too late.

The doctor was charged with abusing his license to prescribe but was acquitted – he claimed to frequently give Elvis placebos and was trying to reduce his drugs. 12 years later the case was reopened and his license was revoked. In 2009 he held an auction of Elvis's prescription pill bottles, with original pills inside.

Dr Nick wasn't the only doctor Elvis managed to get prescriptions from. He studied the Physicians' Desk Reference and would visit other doctors and fake symptoms in order to get more prescriptions.

He was admitted to rehab twice, allegedly for exhaustion, but actually because he had overdosed.

Friends reported that Elvis – always impetuous – became increasingly unpredictable and paranoid. They knew he was experimenting with pain medication but he refused to listen when they tried to help.

The other huge problem was his obesity. Many years after Elvis's death, a journalist reported that:

> *'Presley has become a grotesque caricature of his sleek, energetic former self. Hugely overweight, his mind dulled by the pharmacopoeia he daily ingested, he was barely able to pull himself through his abbreviated concerts.'*

The drugs probably didn't help his weight, messing with his metabolism and keeping him in an almost comatose state at times, but there was another huge cause – his well-known over-eating.

His life-long love of southern cooking – fried, deep fried, and re-fried foods – was a big problem. He took it further though and, instead of enjoying the food, he ate so much of it that he must surely have been unable to enjoy it, it must have been more like a feeding frenzy followed by pain and bloating – and yet more constipation..

Just as Elvis insisted that he needed the drugs to keep up his energy for performing and then sleep afterwards, he used food in the same way. Not as fuel but as medication.

Elvis's cook for 14 years, Mary Jenkins Langston[41], once told a documentary-maker:

> *[Elvis] said that the only thing in life he got any enjoyment out of was eating.'*

How sad. His talent didn't bring him happiness, neither did his achievements, his money, his family, or his friends. Only food. But at least he did get plenty of that so he did have some enjoyment!

Elvis died in his bathroom, a place where he spent a lot of time due to constipation. His autopsy report makes interesting and very sad reading. His heart and liver were twice the size that would be expected of a man his age. His hair, under the dye, was completely white. It took several men to lift his colon out of his body. It was

---

[41] She had started at Graceland as a maid, but Priscilla promoted her to cook.

almost solid, caked with the build-up of many years of overeating and poor food choices. No wonder he suffered so badly from constipation, it must have been very painful and debilitating.

What We Can Learn From Elvis

PRESCRIPTION DRUGS ARE STILL DRUGS

Elvis was against drugs but only illegal drugs. He remained convinced to his death that drugs prescribed by doctors were safe. We know today that many people are killed every year by 'safe' prescription drugs: by over-use; by self-medicating; by 'off-label' use; and by allergic reactions. All drugs come with their dangers.

We know that Elvis took speed to give him energy, diet pills to try to control his weight, and sleeping tablets to help him sleep. He also took medications for various afflictions, including his severe digestive problems and his blood pressure. The combination of all these drugs altered him tremendously – physically and mentally. For such an attractive man to become so overweight must have been dreadful and would have affected his self-esteem and energy. So he took more drugs to help. It was a vicious, fatal circle.

At the time of writing, a University of Washington study[42] about antihistamines is in the news. The simple tablets that we take when the pollen is high, that also

---

[42] http://sop.washington.edu/higher-dementia-risk-linked-use-common-drugs

help us sleep, are causing quite a scare as the study linked their prolonged or high dose use to dementia.

The study proved:

> *"A significantly increased risk for developing dementia, including Alzheimer's disease, to taking commonly used medications with anticholinergic effects at higher doses or for a longer time."*
>
> Dr Shelly Gray et. All, University of Washington/Group Health study

These tablets that we can buy so easily, that many of us carry in our purses, are linked to a dreadful degenerative disease. Now, we don't have to be needlessly scared. The study pointed out that the risk is only there for people who take the older, sedating type of antihistamines, in high doses, every day for over three years. They say it is unlikely that people need antihistamines all year, only when the pollen count is high.

The problem is that, because these tablets are so readily available, people think they are completely safe. So they take them all year round to help them sleep, or to get rid of itching, or other reasons.

A drug is a drug, whether it is from a dealer, a doctor, or a drugstore. They all have their risks and we are all better off with as few of them in our bodies as possible.

It's a good idea to review all medicines and even supplements that you take every few months. Your doctor may not know that you take a whole load of vitamins and minerals – and he/she needs to know because it affects what you can be prescribed.

DON'T LEAVE HEALTH PROBLEMS UNTREATED

Overeating can be a sign of something else – not necessarily a mental health problem but a sign that something else isn't right. A full checkup by a physician is a good idea. Blood tests can reveal nutrient deficiencies and other things that can be put right very easily (and cheaply).

It is worth considering emotional issues as well, as overeating is called 'comfort' eating for a reason. Many of us (me included!) self-medicate with food when we are stressed or anxious. It sounds trivial but food is potent medication.

Foods that are naturally rich in tryptophan (an amino acid) have sedating effects, as do carbohydrates. Amino acids (the building blocks of protein) are also interesting. In the US they are classed as dietary supplements but in Europe and Canada they are thought of as drugs.

> *There is no clear delineation between*
> *a food and a drug.*
>
> Nutritional Neuroscience

IF YOU LOVE SOUTHERN STYLE COOKING KEEP IT FOR SPECIAL OCCASIONS

Elvis's bodyguards said he started using speed and diet pills at the height of his career to keep his weight down to counteract all the over-eating, and to keep his energy up.

Heavy meals bring on lethargy, it's not surprising that Elvis would try to find something to get his energy up. He could have done it by eating more simply, more cleanly and not sedating himself with carbs and sugars.

Southern cooking is wonderful – at Thanksgiving and other specific occasions. Eaten all the time it is a heart attack waiting to happen. Many amazing southern recipes can be adapted to less greasy and artery-clogging.

GO EASY ON THE SALT

Elvis was fond of salt – very fond. It was the major cause of his bloated facial features. A high salt diet can cause high blood pressure, which can bring on heart disease.

Not only that, but regular salt – 'table' salt – is a particularly nasty concoction with, often, a lot of added chemicals. It is harsh and unhelpful to the body, causing it to retain fluid. Many experts believe table salt is a modern curse, contributing to many illnesses.

We do need real salt, especially when sweating, which Elvis did on stage. The trouble is that we get a taste for salt and then don't enjoy food without it.

To get over a high salt intake, try cutting down gradually and including more naturally sodium-rich foods in your diet while reducing foods that have cheap table salt added to them.

Foods to avoid:

- Peanuts, chips, packaged snacks
- Processed meat
- Sauces and packed mixes
- Some breads
- Fast foods
- Highly processed products – basically anything that comes in a packet!

Foods to include:

- Celery
- Seaweed
- Beetroot
- Cantaloupe
- Spinach

You can have salt on your food, especially if you live in a hot climate, but chose good sea salt over refined table salt - Celtic salt and pink Himalayan salt are good choices. They contain trace minerals that actually help, not hinder, hydration, as well as electrolytes, enzyme enhancers, and other trace elements.

You can find out more about Himalayan and Celtic salt benefits on the Dr Axe website:

http://draxe.com/10-benefits-celtic-sea-salt-himalayan-salt

Other Big People

I studied the lives of several people who's stories didn't make it into the final manuscript of this book, for various reasons. But I thought I'd give them a mention, because their lives mattered and they all have something to teach us.

Richard Griffiths

Richard Griffiths - who played Mr Dursley in the Harry Potter movies - grew up in a traumatized and sad home. He described his childhood as 'loathesome'. His parents were both deaf and were unable to talk. Richard remembered his parents wordless but noisy rows, when they would just scream at each other. The fights sometimes degenerated into physical violence, which he witnessed.

The sadness in the home wasn't just due to his parents'

deafness or their other problems, poverty and debt. They had lost a baby girl, as a result of an accident in hospital, before Richard's birth. His mother had fallen asleep with the baby in her arms and had woken to find her lying dead on the floor. She believed a nurse must have taken her and dropped her – but Richard's father never believed that and it was a lifelong source of conflict between them.

This was enough to set Richard up for eating and health problems but in fact he wasn't a big eater. He later became huge though, despite being very thin as a child.

It was his lack of weight when young that was the problem. The family's physician recommended radiation therapy to help Richard gain weight – which it did. It damaged his pituitary gland, which caused him to gain massive amounts of weight and never lose them.

He died from complications following heart surgery aged 65.

The Buddha

I was all set to delve into the Buddha's life and looked forward to it. I figured his weight was probably caused by social eating, as a lot of modern ministers and pastors understand – it's hard to refuse food from well-meaning members of the congregation!

In fact, the Buddha himself was slim and never had a weight problem. The little Buddha statues don't depict the real Buddha.

According to the website *Daily Buddhism*, the statues are quite a recent thing and are based on a 6th century Chinese Zen monk called Hotei. Hotei was a deity of contentment and abundance.

The original Buddha was Siddhattha Gotama. He was a prince who left his privileged lifestyle to live in the wilderness for six years. He was very thin due to that experience. When he returned to civilization, he lived a 'Middle Path', without extremes – and that included eating or drinking too much or too little. He also wasn't bald and didn't expose his belly. So many misconceptions abound about him – but I think that's quite normal, sadly, for many religious leaders.

JOHN CANDY

The towering Canadian actor with the boyish face and fun personality was actually very shy. He made light of his size but hurt inside. He spoke to an interviewer about his size:

> *'I'm the one who has to look in the mirror. And after a while it begins to eat at you.'*

He went to personal trainers and tried numerous diets – including crash diets - but ultimately he was on a road to self-destruction. He believed he had inherited early-death genes from his father, who died from heart problems. John felt it didn't matter what he did or didn't do himself, he was doomed to suffer from the same problems as his father.

Such a fatalistic outlook was bound to have a huge effect on him. It stopped him eating and living healthily – he smoked a pack of cigarettes a day and was known to dabble in drugs.

He loved cooking and entertaining friends at gargantuan feasts.

He suffered badly from anxiety and, like many others, used food to help that. One of his friends, producer Peter Kaminsky commented on John's panic attacks:

> *'He would just stand backstage before he went on with his eyes shut, breathing in and out. Eating, ingesting, smoking, for John it was a way of swallowing that anxietyError! Bookmark not defined..'*

John died, unexpectedly, of a heart attack aged just 43.

WINSTON CHURCHILL

The well-known leader of England during World War II was overweight because he was a foodie - he just ate a lot. He also enjoyed alcohol – but good alcohol. He told a member of staff:

> *'If you want to get drunk, do get drunk on something decent.'*

For his size, though, he was surprisingly healthy. His blood pressure was 140/80 when he was in his 80s, in spite of his regular drinking and cigar smoking.

He claimed to require alcohol before, during, and after meals but he was rarely seen drunk. He did have a glass of Scotch whiskey on hand at all times but it was very, very dilute – mostly water. One member of staff called it more of a mouthwash than a drink.

The reasons for him remaining healthy are that he ate good food, not processed food ('I am only satisfied with the best,' he said), he drank most of his alcohol with food, and he rarely smoke more than a third of a cigar.

NORVELL 'OLIVER' HARDY

Oliver Hardy had a big appetite from his first bite of food. He was obese even as a child and was around 250lbs at the height of his fame. Taunts from other children just spurred him into comedy, as he realized he could make them laugh with him instead of at him.

The loss of his confederate veteran father (before Hardy turned one) and his brother, in an accident, may have contributed to his eating problems. The fact that he changed his name to Oliver, like his father, is significant.

He was difficult at school and his mother sent him to military college. He wasn't interested in lessons but did join a theatrical group.

Hardy took up golf in his teens and played his whole

life. It may have helped him live longer than he would have done without an active hobby.

He grew larger after retiring from acting, going up to 350lbs. He was also a lifelong smoker.

What did make him ill was a crash diet late in his life, which brought on numerous health problems. He lost over 150lbs in just a few months.

His last year was horrible, as a stroke rendered him speechless. When his former partner Stan visited, they did manage to communicate using mime and mimicry. He died aged 65, after whispering 'I love you' to his wife.

ॐ

Sad stories and there are plenty of other people I haven't covered. Other kings, queens, and country leaders, politicians, celebrities, and, of course, people like us. People whose lives aren't played out on the public stage – thankfully! Can you imagine the agony of seeing yourself on your worst day plastered on the front of the *National Enquirer*?!

You would think that these people had all the resources in the world at their disposal, and all the reasons they could have needed to spur them on to lose weight. They did. They could afford the best foods, trainers, exercise systems, and motivational coaches. But they couldn't make permanent weight loss and good health part of their lives.

So how can we expect to? Well, things are a bit different

now. We know a lot more about nutrition, how hormones affect weight, and how psychology can be used in our favor. Let's delve into that...

Part 3

Weight-Loss
In Our Time

Why Some People
Stay Slim

Researching and writing this book has given me a small insight into the sometimes tragic lives of the people featured in these pages. Without exception, they had reasons for their weight problems – reasons that weren't their fault.

There's so much fat-shaming today. Obese people are reviled and their shamers assume that obesity is a very simple self-control issue.

People still believe that to lose weight, the obese just need to move more and eat less. But it is so much more complicated than that.

The people whose lives I studied for this book did that – they embarked on very restrictive diets and they exercised (Elvis performed night after night in energetic shows under hot lights that rivaled the effects of any sauna). But, even when they did lose weight – lots of weight – it came back.

It has proved to me that weight gain and loss are so much more than simple calorie control and exercise. There are always other issues, other things going on when there is a chronic weight problem. No one thing seems to cause it, it can be anything from childhood abuse, poverty, rejection, ill-health, an accident, or a divorce.

What I realized was that the people who really suffer are those who don't find *other* ways of coping with whatever their issues are. Those who do find ways of coping (that don't involve stress/comfort eating) tend to stay slim and active.

Take Elizabeth I, for instance, the virgin queen who gave her name to the colony of Virginia. She was Henry VIII's daughter so genetically disposed towards being overweight, we would assume. But in fact she had a very good figure, even into old age. She was known for her long, slim fingers and would show them off at any opportunity. The Lady Chapel at Westminster Abbey in London houses her effigy. It depicts the queen in old age – still slim. One of her corsets survives and it shows that she had a very slim waist.

How did she manage that? She suffered from the same pressures of leadership as her father, she shared some personality traits, she had a similar heartache in that she wasn't leaving a male heir (or any heir in her case), she had similar abundant food choices put in front of her every day. And she almost certainly never did a sit up or side bend in her life. Why didn't she balloon physically like Henry did?

I believe the answer lies in the way she dealt with things – her coping strategies. She faced many problems in her early life:

- ➢ Losing her mother at a young age.
- ➢ Losing her royal titles and privilege.
- ➢ Being at risk of her life when her sister gained the throne.
- ➢ Being locked up in prison, with the possibility of execution hanging over her.
- ➢ Losing the love and trust of her beloved step-mother Catherine Parr due to having an illicit relationship with Catherine's husband (which may or may not have been consensual).

And then, later on, when she was queen:

- ➢ Having to have her royal cousin put to death because she was a threat to Elizabeth's throne.
- ➢ Pressure from politicians and advisors, who pressured her to marry when she didn't want to.
- ➢ Finding herself an enemy of Spain and facing an expensive war she could well have lost.

Endless problems – more than many of us today will ever face, but some were surprisingly similar to some of our modern issues:

- ➢ **You have financial problems, difficulty meeting your rent/mortgage/loans?** *Elizabeth had an entire country's debt to deal with. It put her and the country in danger and fear of war (which was very expensive).*

➢ **People have rejected you?** *Elizabeth knew rejection. She was declared illegitimate by her own father, plotted against by the head of a religion (the Pope, who called her the 'pretended queen of England and servant of crime' and encouraged members of the Roman Catholic church to take up 'weapons of justice' against her)*

➢ **You have relationship difficulties?** *Elizabeth outlived her siblings and parents at a young age; she had religious differences with her father and sister; she spent most of her reign resisting advisors who wanted her to marry; she was unable to wed the love of her life (political reasons) and had to keep her true relationship with him secret; she also had a very uneasy relationship with her cousin, Mary Queen of Scots, who kept trying to take Elizabeth's throne – in the end, against all her own principles, she had to agree to Mary's execution.*

➢ **You suffered from abuse or neglect as a child?** *Not to belittle your experience but Elizabeth did go through some stuff. She was neglected emotionally and physically by her father (the woman he put in charge of her household had to write and beg for new clothes for her); she was imprisoned by her sister; and there is more than a hint in the history books that she was sexually abused by her step-mother's new husband (after her father's death).*

➢ **You suffer from pain or had an accident that restricts your mobility?** *Elizabeth lived in a era* *without painkillers. She had frequent severe pain from toothache (which caused gum disease and neuralgia), as well as from a varicose ulcer on her leg (almost the same as her father's). And let's not forget the biggest restriction of all – she lived in an era where women were strapped into tight, uncomfortable corsets every day. Corsets restrict movement and affect breathing. She could hardly go jogging trussed up like that.*

➢ **You have physical deformities?** *Elizabeth contracted the often deadly disease smallpox and was left with facial scars. She covered them with her trademark thick white makeup and set a fashion trend. She was not considered conventionally beautiful, yet she drew men to her with her magnetic personality.*

➢ **You have personality flaws?** *Elizabeth was a little neurotic; she had what we would now recognize as panic attacks; she was vain; and her ministers despaired over her indecision and procrastination. She still rocked as Queen and is considered one of the greatest England ever had.*

➢ **You have lost hope/faith?** *Elizabeth hoped she would make it to become queen but the odds were strongly against her until the very day it happened (after her sister's death) and her life was in danger both before and after the crown was placed on her head. She had a strong faith but it must have been rocked at times as, throughout her life, her country was ravaged by religion – hundreds were put to death because they were not of the* *prevailing denomination, which changed with each monarch. How do you continue to believe when religion seems to be the problem? She managed it, and she put her country back together and allowed people to practice whatever religion they wanted to, as long as it didn't interfere with others' rights.*

How did she manage to cope so well?

With wit and intelligence. With a knowledge of her own natural and studied abilities (flirting, diplomacy, multiple languages). With the ability to seek advice from others when her own skills were lacking. With a no-nonsense attitude and a refusal to give up.

Elizabeth wasn't a lone ranger. She sought out people who could help her. She didn't face the Spanish Armada alone when they came to kill her and take over England – she assembled an army, dressed herself in armor and gave her make-shift soldiers such an incredible speech that it fired them up to crush the Armada.[43]

She also knew when to rely on her own efforts – such as resisting all her advisors when they tried to pressure her to marry. She knew what was best for England: it was her, not some foreign princely usurper.

She wasn't without quite serious flaws and she did make mistakes. But she always bounced back. She developed health coping strategies, not self-destructive

---

[43] In the end, the weather was what really helped win the battle – the tide turned and the Spanish ships were blown off-course and out of formation and easier for the English to attack.

ones.

We can learn a lot from Elizabeth. It has always surprised me that she is known as the 'Virgin Queen' (especially as she had at least two relationships which seem to have involved more than just polite conversation!). The disgrace of her mother's execution, her own royal titles being stripped from her, and the Catholic religion swearing against her right to be queen could have crushed her. They didn't. She was more of a Teflon queen – whatever bad stuff was thrown at her, she let it roll off her.

Elizabeth was a human being, made up of the same type of flesh and blood as you and I. She just made the most of what she had, used whatever resources she had at her disposal, and bluffed her way through the rest!

I can't help wondering what she would be like if she had been born into our era – and what she would do if she found herself gaining weight and unable to lose it.

I think she would surround herself with the best advisors, listen carefully to them, then decide which of their guidance she would follow. Our equivalent is to consult doctors, specialists, natural medicine experts, and weight-loss experts. Or, if funds don't stretch far, slimming clubs, online slimming groups, and informal friendship-based health groups.

Elizabeth was vain enough to not want to gain weight. I would bet that she was wise enough to notice that the larger members of her court were the ones who didn't join in when the court went riding, who lingered longer at dinner, or who drank more alcohol than others. I think she would have noticed that the slimmer people were the ones who led the dancing or who ate more fruits and vegetables instead of fatty meats and pastries.

I don't think she would have been keen to try every headline-grabbing diet or extreme exercise plan. She was too wise to be attracted to the latest trend. She didn't survive so long and so well by jumping from idea to idea. She made her decision (eventually!), stuck with it, and saw it through.

I really don't think she would resort to fasting or detox diets. She played a long game. She would do things day by day to get to her goal and not expect her goal to come quicker just because she was doing more extreme things.

The people who stay slim are not necessarily blessed with naturally good metabolisms. They are the people who have good coping strategies – either inherited, learned, or self-developed.

In our information age we are easily able to surround ourselves with trusted advisors – by checking out reviews online first, not by relying on Dr Google! We can increase our knowledge and develop our skills. We can learn what's good to eat and what's not; what exercise choices there are available to us if we are restricted in some areas; what lifestyle choices are best for us.

We don't have to give in and be fatalistic about our inherited genes, past experiences, accidents, or injuries, poor metabolism, or addictions to food, drink, or drugs.

You and only you are the master of your own body. It's great to take advice but it's also good to go with your gut instinct sometimes.

Trends in health and dieting change frequently. One minute it's all aerobics and going for the burn, the next it's about taking it easy with yoga, and the next it's about short-burst high intensity training.

Only you know what suits you, your body, your temperament and what you will be able to stick to.

Only you will be able to decide to change your mind and your attitude, and to find better coping strategies so that you can become and remain a calm, naturally slim person.

Fat & Sugar – The Dangerous Combination

When my herbalist told me many years ago to avoid fat and sugar combinations I was skeptical. She emphasized the addictive nature of the combination and said she believed that was the cause of obesity for many people.

Then came the anti-fat years, when 'health' foods were marketed as low fat but they contained large amounts of sugar. The short-term results were often good, as people would lose weight but they would often regain more than they lost. That's because we do need oils in our diets and if we go on long-term low fat diets we are depriving our bodies of vital nutrients that they will eventually cause us to crave.

Now we're in the anti-sugar years, when the tide has turned and sugar is the demon weight-wise. Or I should say sugar is the demon again, because I can remember my Dad going on a doctor-led diet back in the 70s that was low sugar/carbohydrate. He lost weight by giving up sugar and severely restricting bread and potatoes - and he never regained that weight.

I'm English and can remember a pamphlet the NHS put out for diabetics years ago. It advised them to eat no more than two potatoes a day. That pamphlet disappeared pretty quickly and was replaced by one which didn't recommend potato restriction. I don't **know** that the English version of the Potato Marketing Board, the Potato Council, had anything to do with it but I'd love to know who the sponsors of the pamphlet were!

The fact is that low sugar diets do work – because in the west we eat so much sugar, especially added and hidden sugars.

Today health experts are teaching the fact that sugar turns off fat burning hormones – and that is true. But that doesn't mean we need to eliminate **natural** sugars completely if we need to lose weight.

As we have seen through this book, the big problem is that people embark on extreme diets, depriving themselves of their favorite foods, and eventually they crack and eat everything in sight. The brain is very powerful and it knows when we need certain nutrients. It will cause unbelievably strong cravings to get us to eat foods that contain those nutrients.

The trouble is that we eat many denatured foods now, foods that are produced in factories with no thought for freshness, vitamins, minerals, trace elements, enzymes, etc. So what the brain believes to be real foods are often fake foods – fast food, cookies that are mostly chemicals, packaged meals – that don't really contain the nutrients the brain is seeking. So the brain gets confused and just keeps the cravings coming.

If you are deficient in essential fatty acids, your brain may prompt you to eat foods that contain fats and, if those foods are not only high fat but are high sugar as well, you will get a pleasure high. The combination of fat and sugar causes the release of several fat *storing* hormones – which you really don't want. So sugar is bad enough because it switches off fat burning hormones, but eating it with fat is even worse because it will actually tell your body to store fat.

The bottom line is that, if you want to lose weight or not put any on, you need to avoid foods that combine high fat and high sugar. That's basically anything baked or that comes out of a factory.

Wean yourself off of packaged high fat/high sugar foods by switching to small quantities of natural high fat/high sugar foods. Natural foods have the advantage of coming wrapped up with fiber and the nutrients needed to digest them. Try:

➢ Sliced apple spread or dipped with peanut or almond butter.

➢ Coconut oil mixed with cacao powder and a little natural sweetener (coconut sugar, honey, molasses, maple syrup) to make raw chocolate that is more delicious than the real thing. It just has to be kept refrigerated.

> ➢ Baked chips made by finely slicing potatoes and/or other root vegetables (sweet potatoes and beets are excellent), tossing them in good quality oil (olive or coconut), and sprinkling them with Celtic or Himalayan salt. Either bake them or dehydrate them until they are crisp.

Why Going Hungry Doesn't Work

Many people think they need to run on empty, because that will make their body release fat from the stores. Initially that may happen, if all the other things are in place with fat releasing hormones being on and fat storing hormones being off.

However, what happens when we regularly go hungry is that a hormone called ghrelin is released. Ghrelin is a hunger hormone, it appears when we go without food, in an effort to get us to eat again. Ghrelin causes cravings for this perfect storm of the fat and sugar combination. When we give into that we get addicted to it and we get bigger and bigger. As we can see from most of the chapters in this book.

Weight loss expert and naturopath Dr Jade Teta says on her website, MetabolicEffect[44]:

---

[44] http://www.metaboliceffect.com/worst-food-combination-for-weight-loss

> *'Ghrelin should probably be called the yo-yo weight gain hormone, and those who practice eating less and exercising more are unwittingly raising their ghrelin and fat storing potential.'*

Ghrelin is a problem for dieters who think that they need to go hungry in order to lose weight. In fact, we need to return to regular eating habits and nourish our bodies in order to lose weight healthy and permanently. Lots of overweight people firmly believe that they will be healthy only after they have lost weight – yet the complete opposite is true. We need to get healthy in order to lose weight.

When we don't eat enough, or eat regularly, our systems get messed up. Our metabolism gets confused, our pancreas starts getting trigger happy pumping out insulin at the drop of a hat, and our brain thinks there's a war on and that's why there isn't enough food coming in. At the potential famine to come, the brain will cause cravings, to get more fat in the stores to survive the trouble to come.

That's why people who do strict diets find that, once they return to 'normal' eating, they pile more weight on than before. The body thinks another famine is coming and it needs to lay down stores.

In the old days of agricultural living, when people had to grow or hunt their own food, this was a valuable survival mechanism. In times of food shortage, as many people as possible would survive, because they had enough stored in their fat cells to carry them through. Then, once there was more to eat, their bodies could lay down new fat stores ready for the next shortage.

Most of us don't have problems of feast or famine now though. Food surrounds us, in stores, in homes, at social events, at work. Too much is the problem more than too little. Yet the body still operates the feast or famine response. So when we don't eat enough it tries to keep as much as possible and put it into the fat stores.

So we can see that depriving the body of food isn't a great idea. It sets us up for the yo-yo dieter's nightmare and can really mess with our metabolisms.

A friend of mine was ill with anorexia some years ago and went to stay with relatives who lived on a farm. She helped with the cows, horses, chickens, fencing, and everything else. She ate everything put in front of her! She was hungry because she was active, doing hard physical work.

When she returned home she wasn't doing all that work anymore but she could still eat as much without putting weight on, because she had broken the feast or famine cycle that her body had got into. It no longer mistrusted her and thought there was a war on with food shortages – it knew food was coming. So her metabolism returned to normal. As she was eating regularly, she had more energy and was able to return to her favorite sports, walk her dog, and do other normal activities – whereas before, when she had hardly been eating, she had had no energy to do anything.

Breaking The Vicious Cycle Is The Key

My friend broke the vicious cycle with food and activity. Note that I didn't say exercise – which can be a turn-off to many people thanks to school Physical Ed lessons! Activity, hobbies, sports, spending time in nature, loving movement, doing stuff, getting the sofa off your back, whatever you want to call it, it helps break the cycle.

Henry VIII piled weight on after having to give up jousting – he gave up all exercise and took up comfort eating. What a pity he didn't take up a less violent sport instead, which would have been good stress relief and not caused him to use food as a self-prescribed drug.

The current obesity epidemic coincided with the decline of families sitting down to eat together and eating three meals a day at regular times. Instead, we are all busy and tend to grab food on the run more times than we'd care to admit to!

As more and more of us work long and unsocial hours, family mealtimes have been replaced with feeding the children separately, the adults eating together later so they can have a bit of calm, and lots of meals eaten behind the steering wheel of a car or at a desk. We also tend to skip meals.

There are a lot of advantages to returning to a more regular way of eating – in whatever way that works for each of us.

When our body knows that food is coming in a couple of hours, it isn't going to cause us to crave things. It isn't going to cause trouble, it will just wait quietly.

Regular mealtimes, with others if possible, prevent us from binging (others notice!). They prevent us from needing midnight snacks. They are a form of stress relief – if you can take meals with relaxing people, that is!

Families talk about their days over dinner, the children get to release stress by bringing up things that bothered them at school, parents get to talk over issues at work or financial struggles. Talking is a form of stress relief and talking around a dinner table has a primeval nurturing effect. Same as it ever was. Your grandparents discussed their day over dinner – and their day possibly included real wars, times of financial depressions, and other difficulties.

Unhappiness seems to me to be one of the biggest causes of weight problems. Just look at the people featured in this book. In every single case, their weight problems were caused or made worse by unhappiness.

A quote I love from *Jurassic Park* can be applied to people who pursue weight-loss above all else, even at the extent of their health:

> *'They don't have intelligence. They have what I call 'thintelligence'. They see the immediate situation. They think narrowly and they call it 'being focused'. They don't see the surround. They don't see the consequences.'*
>
> Ian Malcolm, *Jurassic Park*

Many of the people featured in this book were very focused on losing weight. They were able to endure strict fasting or calorie restricting diets, they weren't short of willpower or reasons to lose weight. But they didn't see the bigger picture. They wanted quick short-term results, they didn't consider their long-term health.

Then, when the diet no longer seemed to be working (i.e. their brain assumed there was a famine and started holding onto fat reserves), their cravings got too powerful, or stress overwhelmed them, they returned to their old eating habits, their old ways of coping.

When I went through a bad period of depression following an accident, a therapist told me that depression was caused by a feeling of not being in control and to find some little thing – anything – that I could control.

The loss of control feeling is one that affects many illnesses, not just mild depression but severe, clinical depression and many types of eating and anxiety disorders. We go downhill when we feel like there's nothing we can do to help ourselves or alter our situation, if the situation is bad.

Unfortunately, many of us choose coping strategies that are self-destructive. The anorexic who feels her life spiraling out of control and who finds that she feels powerful and proud of her willpower when she can resist hunger will cling on to that feeling as the only thing that makes her feel better – until it kills her.

There is always something constructive we can do. Even if we can't do anything physically (such as magic up more money if we're dreadfully in debt), we can do something with our **attitude**.

Attitude is everything. Get that right and everything improves. Get it wrong and everything not only seems worse, it actually gets worse. That's because a bad attitude attracts bad events like manure attracts flies.

Have you ever seen those little toy cars that stop when they bump into things then change direction and go trundling off again, just as fast as before? A good attitude is like that.

Life will cause us to bump into relationship and job roadblocks, brick walls, financial potholes. Our attitude is what makes us change direction when we need to and keep going when things get tough.

As another famous line in the film *Jurassic Park* goes:

> **'Life will find a way.'**

Your brain and your body are magnificent – whatever shape you're in. Your brain is more powerful than the most high-spec computer ever created, your body more adaptable than

If we keep looking for positive coping strategies, life will find a way.

The people in this book all wanted to find quick ways of solving their weight problems. They wanted to look and feel better NOW. We all do. But it simply doesn't work.

What does work is small, consistent life changes. Losing a lot of weight in a short space of time puts an incredible strain on the organs, and most people who lose a lot of weight put it back on again – unless they change their lifestyle generally.

Perhaps you want to lose weight for an event, or so you can wear summer clothes without wanting to hide in a muumuu. That's why people do desperate things, try extreme diets. Then it doesn't work and they go right back to their regular eating habits.

There will be other events, there will be other sunny days. Time will pass anyway, you may as well spend it by making small changes that will improve your health generally and reduce your weight gradually.

I strongly recommend only taking up one new habit or lifestyle change at once. Otherwise you can get overwhelmed and give you.

So do one small thing – perhaps drinking a glass of water first thing in the morning – and keep that up for 10 days before adding an additional thing. When you are feeling good, you can think about cutting out one bad thing – perhaps replacing a soda habit with a sparkling water habit, or starting to bake cookies with reduced sugar rather than buying them (check the ingredients, if sugar is in the first three ingredients there's too much of it in there!)

If you already do lots of healthy things and just can't

understand why you can't lose weight, it may be worth seeing a naturopathic doctor. You could have a food intolerance or an underlying health issue.

Pulse Testing

I was introduced to pulse testing by my herbalist and it helped me understand occasional bouts of indigestion, abdomen pain, and diarrhea. Once I started really taking it seriously, it also helped my general health.

Pulse Testing has bad reputation among medical professionals, who associate it with what they think of as quack doctors. They have a point, as it can be very dangerous to use it for full-on food allergies without the attention of a medical professional.

It is generally associated with a medical doctor, American allergist, Dr Arthur Coca, who came up with it as a way to identify problem foods for his patients.

The idea is that the body has to deal with every food we eat, breaking it down and processing it. When we eat foods that we are intolerant to, our hearts beat faster and our pulses rise.

So we need to find out which foods make our pulse rise.

If you do this, be sure to only test foods that don't cause you to have extreme reactions. If you know you can't eat, say, strawberries, don't be tempted to eat some just to see if they make your pulse rise! Real food allergies are extremely serious. This is just to find out minor reactions.

Pulse testing is safe and easy to do at home but it takes a few days to get the best, most accurate results.

Pulse Testing Stage One

For several days, take your pulse at the following times and make a note of the numbers and times:

- ➢ Before getting out of bed, just after waking up
- ➢ Before each meal
- ➢ After each meal
- ➢ Just before going to sleep

I have included a worksheet you can use for your notes. Also write down what you ate and any changes in your feelings throughout the time of the testing period.

Some experts recommend taking the pulse for 30 seconds, other for a minute. Whichever you choose, stick to that for the duration of the testing.

This first stage gives you an idea of what your pulse is generally. You may notice that it tends to rise a little after you eat or drink anything, or you may start to spot patterns where it rises more significantly after certain foods. This could be a reaction to something in those foods, which we'll delve into next.

Pulse Testing Stage Two

Start testing individual foods – as simple as possible. Test an onion rather than an onion bhaji, or an apple rather than apple pie.

> ➢ Sit down comfortably and relax for 10 minutes
> ➢ Put a little piece of a simple food on your tongue (don't swallow yet!)
> ➢ Take your pulse
> ➢ Swallow the food
> ➢ Take your pulse again at 2 minute intervals, 3 more times[45]

If your pulse rises by three or more beats, your body is showing signs of stress towards that food. If it rises more significantly, and/or stays raised, you may have a more serious intolerance. It would be a good idea to make an appointment to see an allergist.

---

[45] Some practitioners go further and test again 30, 60, and 90-minute intervals. I've never had the patience to do that!

Bibliography

Bauso, T. (1994). Mother Knows Best: The Voices of Mrs Bates in Psycho. *Hitchcock Annual.*

Brando, Turner Classic Movies [Motion Picture].

Brooks, M. (n.d.). *Celebrities | Mel Brooks.* Retrieved 2014, from Bon Appetit:
http://www.bonappetit.com/people/celebrities/article/
mel-brooks-on-omelettes-coffee-and-the-inimitable-
appetite-of-alfred-hitchcock

Costandi, M. (2006). *The Psychology of Alfred Hitchcock.*
Retrieved November 2014, from NeuroPhilosophy:
http://neurophilosophy.wordpress.com/2006/10/17/the
-psychology-of-alfred-hitchcock

Fawell, J. (2004). *Hitchcock's Rear Window.* Southern Illinois University Press.

Fiegel, E. (2006). *Dream a Little Dream of Me: The Life of 'Mama' Cass Elliot.* Pan.

Green, D. B. (2014, December). This Day in Jewish History / Singer Cass Elliot.

Gregg, E. (2001). *Queen Anne.* Yale University Press.

Guralnick, P. (2014). *Last Train to Memphis: The Rise of Elvis Presley.* Little, Brown and Company.

Buddha, K. (2011). *Brain over Binge.* Camellia Publishing, LLC.

Harding, J. (2012, January 27). *A right royal catfight.* http://www.dailymail.co.uk/home/books/article-2092313/A-right-royal-catfight-QUEEN-ANNE-THE-POLITICS-OF-PASSION-BY-ANNE-SOMERSET.html

Kings and queens - The Stuarts - 1603-1714. (n.d.). History of England: http://www.historyofengland.net/kings-and-queens/the-stuarts-1603-1714-background#

Lewis, J. (1789). *Memoirs of Prince William Henry, Duke of Gloucester.*

Lieberman, H. R., Kanarek, R. B., & Prasad, C. (2005). *Nutritional Neuroscience.* CRC Press.

McKittrick, C. (2014). *Fellows Find: How Hollywood Producers Used Alfred Hitchcock's Weight To Their Advantage.* Cultural Compass: http://blog.hrc.utexas.edu/2013/12/02/fellows-find-hitchcocks-weight/

Murgatroyd, C. (n.d.). *Blood Disorders - Porphyria.* Retrieved 2014, from Power Of The Gene: http://powerofthegene.com/joomla/index.php/genetically-inherited-diseases/blood-disorders/porphyria

Norton Greenberger, R. V. (2009). *4 Weeks to Healthy Digestion: A Harvard Doctor's Proven Plan for Reducing Symptoms of Diarrhea, Constipation, Heartburn & More.* McGraw-Hill.

Peele, S. (1986). *Personality, Pathology, and The Act of Creation: The Case of Alfred Hitchcock*. Retrieved 2014, from The Stanton Peele Addiction Website: http://www.peele.net/lib/hitch.html

Somerset, A. (2013). *Queen Anne: The Politics of Passion*. Random House.

Spoto, D. (2009). *Spellbound by Beauty: Alfred Hitchcock and his Leading Ladies*. Three Rivers Press.

Wilson, B. (2013, January 25). *Alfred Hitchcock's complicated relationship with food*. Retrieved November 2014, from The Telgraph: http://www.telegraph.co.uk/journalists/bee-wilson/9818987/Alfred-Hitchcocks-complicated-relationship-with-food.html

Winn, J. A. (2014). *Queen Anne: Patroness of Arts*. Oxford University Press.

Footnotes/Additional Sources

1. http://channel.nationalgeographic.com/channel/episodes
   inside-the-body-of-henry-viii
2. It was a good match in many ways as Elizabeth was a Plantagenet, the old dynasty. It helped heal the wounds of war and unite two dynasties.
3. http://journals.ed.ac.uk/resmedica/article/viewFile/403/684
4. https://suite.io/tracey-white/5qzy2nv
5. http://youtu.be/fCbZ60q9NYo
6. http://draxe.com/why-you-should-avoid-pork/
7. http://www.dailymail.co.uk/health/article-

371528/Halle-Berry-My-battle-diabetes.html

8. James was actually James I of England and VI of Scotland!

9. Historians can't agree on the number of Anne's pregnancies. It varies between 17 and 19, according to who you read!

10. http://powerofthegene.com/joomla/index.php/convers ational-genetics/genetics-in-legends-and-folklaw

11. http://www.ucsfhealth.org/education/substance_use_d uring_
pregnancy

12. http://amzn.com/0992960908 (Shameless plug - I wrote a book on dry skin brushing – but only because it gives such amazing, quick results!)

13. The Bush family have done rather well from their membership too!

14. Beef steak

15. http://blog.hrc.utexas.edu/2013/12/02/fellows-find-hitchcocks-weight

16. http://www.bonappetit.com/people/celebrities/article /mel-brooks-on-omelettes-coffee-and-the-inimitable-appetite-of-alfred-hitchcock

17. http://www.dailymail.co.uk/news/article-2182804/Hitchcock-star-Tippi-Hedren-says-director-evil-shed-rich-sexual-harassment-laws-applied-1960s.html

18. The interview took place before *Psycho* was released. Hitch referred to it as a 'rather gentle horror' that he was planning.
http://the.hitchcock.zone/wiki/Desert_Island_Discs_%2 8BBC_Radio,_19/Oct/1959%29_-_Alfred_Hitchcock

19. Interview on the Mike Douglas Show

20. Mama Cass confirmed a rumor that her vocal range increased after a concussion but this may have been to cover up the fact that John felt she was too fat to join the band.

21. When asked if she had a childhood nickname, Cass said

it was 'Cookie' (the Mike Douglas show interview)

22. http://www.newspapers.com/newspage/17984687
23. http://www.dennydoherty.com/dream/dream18.html
24. The official cause was 'fatty myocardial degeneration due to obesity '.
25. http://www.unm.edu/~lkravitz
26. A pulse test is useful for determining which foods your body reacts to in some way but it isn't a medical test. Don't rely on it to tell you about a food *allergy*. Food allergies can be life-threatening and only proper medical tests are reliable at uncovering them.
27. http://sleepfoundation.org/ask-the-expert/stress-and-insomnia
28. http://www.hsph.harvard.edu/obesity-prevention-source/
obesity-causes/sleep-and-obesity
29. https://justgetflux.com
30. http://www.manythings.org/voa/people/Marlon_Brando.html
31. http://www.lifetimetv.co.uk/biography/biography-marlon-brando
32. http://www.todayifoundout.com/index.php/2012/11/the-odd-eating-habits-of-marlon-brando
33. http://www.chimesdesign.com/blog/2012/04/15/on-binging-and-brando
34. *Somebody*, Stefan Kanfer
35. http://larrykinglive.blogs.cnn.com/2009/06/29/lkl-web-exclusive-michael-jacksons-friend-and-marlon-brandos-son-on-the-michael-jackson-he-knew
36. He like his surname to be pronounced the southern way, PRESSley, not PREZley. Vernon actually spelled his name Pressley until after Elvis became famous.
37. A small, narrow home, similar to a railroad apartment, usually around 12ft wide. They were popular house styles from the end of the Civil War to the 1920s but became symbols of poverty.
38. Constipation was a big problem but even Elvis's doctor

didn't realize how big of a problem until too late.

39. She had started at Graceland as a maid, but Priscilla promoted her to cook.

40. http://sop.washington.edu/higher-dementia-risk-linked-use-common-drugs

41. http://www.metaboliceffect.com/worst-food-combination-for-weight-loss

42. In the end, the weather was what really helped win the battle – the tide turned and the Spanish ships were blown off-course and out of formation and easier for the English to attack.

43. Some practitioners go further and test again 30, 60, and 90-minute intervals. I've never had the patience to do that!

Acknowledgements

I'm told it is considered bad form in the publishing world to have an acknowledgements section that is longer than one page. It is entirely in character and in keeping with the rest of my life for me to have a two-page acknowledgements section!

Much of this book was researched and written while staying at one of my favorite hotels. The Holiday Inn Express at Hemel Hempstead in England has a great pool and gym and is close to London for research (and sight-seeing!). I loved having the pool available to work off stress and knotted muscles. Thanks to the great staff for their hospitality and for picking up after me.

This book would not have been completed without my editor Anna. Huge thanks and sorry for the delay! Thanks to my sister-in-law and fellow author Lynn – it's always great to have someone who understands to talk to. Grateful thanks to Mum & Dad, Josh & Becky, and my fiancé Andrew for their constant support and encouragement.

Special thanks to my high school history teacher for giving me a love of history and for being an animal rights activist. Coolest teacher ever!

Thanks to all at Coo Farm Press for help with this and my previous books.

I really wish the information in this book had been available when my lovely cousin Carolyn 'Lyn' Howard (neé Teare) was alive. Lyn battled weight problems her whole life and died far too young.

I don't know why her weight was such a problem but I have a few ideas, since doing this research. I think stress and hormones were a large part of the mystery – as they are for many of us.

Finally, I'd like to acknowledge everyone who has ever struggled with their weight, who has felt rejected because of it, and who has tried or been tempted to try extreme dieting and other weight-loss measures. You are worth more than what you weigh. You are worth more than what others think of you. Their attitude says far more about them than is does about you.

Keep going.

Mia x

Free Chapter Excerpt from *The 10-Day Skin Brushing Detox*

DEFINITION: ***detox***

A period when you stop taking unhealthy or harmful foods, drinks, or drugs into your body for a period of time, in order to improve your health.

Cambridge Dictionaries

I HAVE CALLED this book a detox plan but this is not like a traditional diet or detox. It isn't the type of detox where you give up lots of your usual food stuffs, suffer a whopping great headache, and spend most of your time groaning in the bathroom.

Detoxification is generally considered to be a removal of toxic substances - often alcohol or drugs. The modern use of the word 'detox' (the shortened term became popular in the 1970s) has been linked with alternative/complementary medicine.

Traditional doctors don't believe in the modern interpretation of the word 'detox' (not to be confused with clinical alcohol/drug detoxification). They don't think there is any need for what health writers call a detox, insisting that the body has its own detoxification organs and processes that don't require additional help.

I don't believe in detoxes either (detoxes where you give up lots of things and suffer from the effects of withdrawal from them, anyway). I don't believe in them because I have tried them and I've seen lots of other people try them and I've found that they don't work, especially long-term. Research has taught me why they don't work.

My plan is simple. It's just 10 days of supporting your body's natural detoxification systems via skin brushing, deep breathing, and rehydrating. Not giving things up, not suffering, and not putting unrealistic expectations on yourself. I have split it into two: one plan for those who are active and in reasonably good health, and one plan for those who are inactive and not in great health.

For both, it is a plan of abundance, not deprivation, because deprivation doesn't work. Deprivation of food - as proved in an experiment during World War II called the Minnesota Starvation Experiment - causes horrendous problems, including:

> ➢ Decreased heart volume.
> ➢ Apathy & depression.
> ➢ Sensitivity to noise.
> ➢ Loss of ambition & narrowing of interests.
> ➢ Increased neuroticism & hysteria.
> ➢ Increased interest & preoccupation with food.
> ➢ Heightened craving for food.
> ➢ Reduction of humor & tolerance.
> ➢ Increased self-centeredness.
> ➢ Inability to control emotions.

Similar to the things a lot of people go through when dieting today.

If you've heard of it at all, you may think that the Minnesota Starvation Experiment involved complete starvation, or fasting. It didn't. The participants merely ate a reduced calorie diet - which contained MORE calories than many modern crash diets – but they weren't sitting around, they were doing some work.

They ate just under half their usual calorie intake for 6 months. This amount was determined by the investigators after observing them eating normally for the previous 3 months.

The Minnesota experiment used volunteers - who were conscientious objectors - to find out what effects famine had on the human body. They needed to know, to determine how to provide relief assistance to famine victims of the war. After the experiment was over it took 33 weeks for the participants to return to normal eating, sleeping, and social behavior and their previous humor 'slowly returned'.

For the sake of clarity, allow me to repeat that. They ate HALF of their usual calories. The volunteers were all healthy men, and their controlled diet caloric intake before the 'starvation' was an average of 3,200 daily (depending on their weight). During the 'starvation' the men ate an average of 1,560 calories each day. **1,560**. That is more than is recommended by many modern diets, a lot more than recommended by some diets (LighterLife recommends just 500-600 calories a day in the initial phase).

The volunteers became obsessed with food during the starvation phase. Their behavior became irrational and uncontrolled. One man actually chopped off three of his fingers with an axe. He later said: "I admit to being crazy mixed up. As of 50 years later, I am not ready to say I did it on purpose. I am not ready to say I didn't."

This sounds like the deliberate self-harm that anorexics go through. Or the passive-aggressive self-harm through drinking, smoking, and drug taking of unhappy models and others who have to remain unnaturally slim.

Do we really want to do this to ourselves? Is a crash diet to lose some weight worth the risk of putting our heart in trouble, alienating friends & family, putting our job security in jeopardy, losing our sense of humor, and more?

The Minnesota experiment produced another effect. Many of the men ended up binging heavily once the experiment was over. Like many of us do when we 'fall off the wagon' when dieting. We swing from starving ourselves to binging and back again. Often, we do this throughout our lives. Perhaps not in as extreme a manner as undergone by the volunteers in the experiment, but if we don't provide our bodies with the calories and nutrients that they need, we will experience the same negative effects, just in a lesser way that takes longer to show the worst of its effects.

The Minnesota experiment demonstrated that people who have endured a period of starvation need up to 5,000 calories a day to recover from it. Not vitamin or protein mixtures, just real food and lots of it. Those of us who have experimented with various diets and detoxes over the years have been responsible for putting ourselves through stress not unlike that suffered by people in war zones. Your body thinks there's a war going on. And you wonder why you're finding it hard to resist food cravings? Your body could be starving for various nutrients and doing whatever it can to get you to eat to get them.

Let's look at what happens when we don't eat enough. Our body will assume something dreadful is happening - such as war or famine (or our agreeing to take part in a starvation experiment!). The body starts to focus on staying alive and won't 'waste' valuable resources (calories/nutrients) on things that aren't essential to life. So no more glossy hair, strong nails, soft skin, bright eyes. And lots of anxiety, depression, loss of concentration, etc.

Many of us live in that state of pseudo famine almost all our lives. Instead of enjoying vibrant health, we have to buy expensive moisturizers to make our faces look less washed out, nail treatments to try to stop our nails flaking and breaking, various drugs and addictions to give us energy (caffeine, sugar) or calm us down enough to be able to sleep (drugs, herbal tranquillizers, other sleep aids - legal and otherwise).

I put it to you that it's time to give your body, your mind, and your spirit a break. It's time to let your body know that you care for it and are going to give it what it needs. Real food. Healthy habits. Care and support.

It's time to let your mind know that you no longer expect it to function on less than adequate nutrition (the brain uses about 300 calories a day - unless it is thinking very hard, when it burns through more); on negative, self-hating thoughts; on stressful, anxious matters.

It's time to let your spirit know that you recognize its existence. You don't have to be religious to acknowledge that you have a spirit.

One last thing before we leave the topic of the Minnesota Starvation Experiment. The main investigator, nutritionist Ancel Keys (who went on to discover the link between cholesterol and heart disease[46]), followed a Mediterranean-type diet - lots of vegetables, olive oil, red wine, fish. That is a diet of abundance and enjoyment. He lived an active life with lots of good food, swimming, and walking. He died at the age of 100 in 2004. He remained a scientist right to the end. Asked at his 100th birthday party if his Mediterranean diet was the reason for his longevity, he said: "Very likely, but no proof."

I found out about Ancel Keys and the Minnesota Starvation Experiment when, in desperation, I took my daughter - who was suffering terribly with the effects of anorexia - to see the well-known UK nutritionist Zoe Harcombe. She sat my daughter in a warm, cozy spot in her kitchen - knowing that anorexics are permanently freezing due to lack of caloric intake. Zoe didn't demand that my daughter explain herself as to why she wasn't eating, knowing that she would be unable to formulate the sentences due to lack of brain food. She just gently told us her own life story, about her battles with anorexia and bulimia and how she overcame them.

She explained about the Minnesota Starvation Experiment and the fact that people need 1,500 calories a day just for basic bodily functions. You need that amount even if you're lying in bed all day, when you add in normal daily activities, work, exercise, study, etc., you need more (much more, in many cases).

My daughter and I realized that, like many other people

---

[46] http://mbbnet.umn.edu/hoff/hoff_ak.html

(women in particular), we had both been putting ourselves through our own mini versions of the Minnesota Starvation Experiment. I had been doing it via various detoxes and diets for over 40 years. My daughter had been doing it via anorexia. Anorexia for her, and for many sufferers, was a crutch to support her through a difficult time. It was her way of coping with something else.

Trying to forcibly remove anorexia is like trying to remove the crutch from a person with one leg, who relies on it for walking. Not a good idea. But when the crutch itself is life-threatening, it's time to find a better crutch, or find a way to do without a crutch completely.

Working with Zoe taught us that we needed to become healthy in order to get better. That might sound like an odd way of putting it but it was a phrase similar to one I heard later on from another of my heroes, Dr Eric Berg, who is a US chiropractor and weight loss expert. He says you shouldn't diet to lose weight, you should get healthy to lose weight. If you aren't healthy enough, your body won't be willing to let go of its emergency food rations that it has so carefully stored in your fat cells.

The story of my life-long battle for health is in Chapter One. If you don't like long stories, you can skip it. I'll put it in a nutshell here:

➢ Years of quite serious ill health after being in a car wreck, followed by multiple surgeries.

> ➤ Yo-yo attempts at dieting, detoxing, and trying to get fit and healthy.

> ➤ Failure and defeat only to try again and fail again - with my weight getting heavier and my health getting worse all the time.

For many years, I was either dieting or binging. When I dieted I was in a state of starvation, of deprivation. When I was off a diet I was in a state of abundance, eating anything I liked, enjoying life. Well, for a while, as eating everything you want makes you feel ill eventually if what you want is unhealthy food!

It's a pretty normal story really. Many people start it every New Year's Eve. We make resolutions to fix the things that have been bothering us. We often do it in such an 'all-or-nothing' way, though, that it is impossible to keep up. Then we give up, defeated, sometime in early January, convincing ourselves that we aren't capable of sticking to anything.

When I discovered a naturopathic technique that had terrific effects, I went at it the way I had done all the diet/health things I tried before - with devastating side-effects. So I gave it up.

Dry skin brushing (I'll call it skin brushing from now on but I always mean brushing that is done with a dry brush on dry skin) is a very simple yet very powerful technique that can be used on its own to improve health, increase lymphatic and blood circulation, tackle cellulite, increase energy, and much more. What it does is give you a glow, a healthy vibrancy that makes you want to eat better and even think better. It helps take you out of the starvation phase of your own personal Minnesota Starvation Experiment and into the recovery phase. The phase of returning to enjoying life, of returning to a healthy weight, of not being obsessed with food or diets or health.

During the recovery phase, the experiment volunteers naturally ate more calories because their bodies knew that the nutrients were needed for rebuilding themselves. After around 15 weeks of eating many more calories than they would have if they hadn't been through the starvation phase, their social behavior started to return to normal. By week 20 they nearly all felt normal around food. By week 33 they had returned to eating normal amounts and no longer binged. Touchingly, the investigators noticed that humor returned.

What does all that have to do with you? Well I imagine that you've been beating up on yourself in one way or another. Perhaps through diets and detoxes, or through negative thinking, exercise (too much or too little of it), alcohol, drugs, overwork. Humans are really creative, we can think of lots of ways to self-destruct!

This little book can help you to stop beating yourself up. It can do that by introducing you to a really quick, easy, effective health technique called skin brushing. Done improperly, though, skin brushing can cause headaches, joint pain, brain fog, nausea, and skin irritation. Those sorts of feelings make you reach for stimulants to make you feel better - caffeine, alcohol, sugar, fats. Once you do, you crave more and it's the old downward spiral to ill-health again.

The definition of detox is a period of giving up harmful things – usually thought to be just food and drinks. Maybe it could also include giving up harmful thoughts too, especially those directed at ourselves.

So I hope you will use the techniques in this book and the advice I heap on in shovelfuls not to take it too quickly or go at it like a bull in a china shop that's located on the way to a field of fertile cows.

Go easy. Go easy on the technique and on yourself. Whatever state you're in, you are actually a work of art, a miracle of biology. For you to have made it through conception, pregnancy, and birth was a fantastic, amazing achievement. Everything else is just detail.

If you enjoyed this excerpt, you can find
***The 10-Day Skin Brushing Detox* on Amazon,**
or you can order it from libraries & bookstores.

Index

N

O

P

If you enjoyed this book or got help from it in any way, please consider leaving a review on Amazon.